# COST MANAGEMENT FOR HOSPITALS

**John G. Nackel, Ph.D.**
Principal
National Office
Ernst & Whinney
Cleveland, Ohio

**George M.J. Kis, CPA**
Senior Manager
National Office
Ernst & Whinney
Cleveland, Ohio

**Paul J. Fenaroli, CPA**
Senior Manager
Ernst & Whinney
Atlanta, Georgia

AN ASPEN PUBLICATION®
Aspen Publishers, Inc.

1987

Rockville, Maryland
Royal Tunbridge Wells

Library of Congress Cataloging-in-Publication Data

Nackel, John G.
Cost management for hospitals.

"An Aspen publication."
Bibliography: p.
Includes index.
1. Hospitals—Business management. 2. Hospital care—
Cost effectiveness. 3. Hospital care—Cost control.
I. Kis, George M. J. II. Fenaroli, Paul J. III. Title.
[DNLM: 1. Cost Benefit Analysis. 2. Economics, Hospital.
3. Hospital Administration. 4. Management Information
Systems. WX 157 N125c]
RA971.3.N33   1987      362.1′1′0681   87-1126
ISBN 0-87189-637-0

Editorial Services: Carolyn Ormes

Library of Congress Catalog Card Number: 87-1126
ISBN: 0-87189-637-0

Printed in the United States of America

1   2   3   4   5

To the health care executives, physicians, and students who promote cost management principles, and to our colleagues at Ernst & Whinney. We hope this book leads to a better understanding and implementation of the ideas presented, to new creative solutions to cost management problems, and to more cost-effective and higher quality health care.

# Contents

# *Foreword*

Cost Management for Hospitals addresses several key changes taking place in health care in the United States today. These changes are themselves reflective of changes in society at large. "Cost efficiency" and "greater productivity" have become watchwords in virtually every sector of American business. The design and implementation of management control systems and industry-specific information systems are some of the principal methods whereby industries attempt to achieve greater efficiency and productivity. This book is a timely discussion of the design and application of such systems as they relate to health care.

Over the last several years, we have observed the transformation of American medicine from a collegial, academically oriented social service into a large, increasingly competitive business. Health care today is being shaped in large measure by changes in payment structures (including cost containment pressures) and the advent of competitive forces heretofore virtually unknown to medicine.

In this new business environment of health care, as in other industries, the prices of goods and services are set and limited, thereby introducing the issues of cost effectiveness and quality and their measurement in a way that has never before been raised. Until recently, those who purchased medical care—third-party payers in particular—made little or no distinction in reference to quality. Insurers basically reimbursed providers at published charges, regardless of any measure of quality. Nor did most of the largest purchasers of health care—the federal government and corporations—make any decisions about limiting or restricting payments to certain providers.

Since about 1980, however, we have begun to see purchasers formulate their health care buying decisions not on the basis of quality, but on the basis of cost. This trend is reflected both in the shift from reimbursement to prospective payment systems and in the significant growth of managed care plans such as health maintenance organizations, preferred provider organizations, and the like.

This, in turn, is having a profound effect on the role of physicians and nurses in regard to cost management and quality assurance. In the past, clinicians were not required to be concerned with the cost of patient care, but only with its quality. The realities of health care today, however, demand that the people who are most directly responsible for resource allocation and utilization—particularly the medical staff—take active roles in managing both cost and quality, tasks for which they traditionally have not been prepared. In Part I, this book provides a welcome foundation to the concept of cost management in a system that is oriented around the patient. This concept gives doctors, nurses, and health care managers a common language in which they can conduct their new responsibilities.

Part II contains information on how to develop a hospital cost management system. In Part III, the authors turn to specific uses and applications of the information derived from a cost management system. How that information is used is critical: It is important to emphasize that while physicians are taking on new responsibilities in the areas of both quality assurance and cost management, they serve dual (and more traditional) roles as patient advocates. There is, perhaps inevitably, a tension between the concept of physician-as-gatekeeper, zealously guarding the portals of the health care system, and physician-as-advocate, who will do whatever he or she "feels" is necessary to care for the patient, regardless of cost.

Clearly, hospitals and the people who work in them must never lose sight of their central mission of providing the best possible care to each patient. The cost management concepts and applications described in these pages give hospitals and clinicians the tools they need to use each available resource in the most cost-efficient, most medically appropriate way. A cost management system is neither designed nor intended to be used for the sole purpose of saving money, but rather as a tool for helping hospitals operate most effectively within the constraints society has imposed.

Jerome H. Grossman, M.D.
Chairman and Chief Executive Officer
New England Medical Center, Inc.

# *Acknowledgments*

Many individuals contributed their thoughts, efforts, and practical experiences toward the realization of this book. To make the book as comprehensive as possible, a group of Ernst & Whinney health care executives from a variety of disciplines shared their time, ideas, and advice. Their collective experience in cost management and their views from different disciplines added considerable value and utility to the text.

My coauthors include George M.J. Kis, an Ernst & Whinney senior manager in our National office, and Paul J. Fenaroli, an Ernst & Whinney senior manager in our Atlanta office. George and Paul relied on their extensive hospital cost management knowledge and experience and supplemented their expertise by working with other Ernst & Whinney health care executives. The other Ernst & Whinney executives who contributed are:

- Joseph J. Alfirevic, Chicago, Illinois
- William L. Caron, Portland, Maine
- David J. Cox, Tampa, Florida
- Thomas J. Crowley, Baltimore, Maryland
- Charles C. Gabbert, Los Angeles, California
- Bruce J. Kronman, Chicago, Illinois
- Richard L. Marrapese, Cleveland, Ohio
- Paul F. McMahon, Cleveland, Ohio
- John E. Moyer, Atlanta, Georgia
- David P. Pfeil, Dallas, Texas
- P. Douglas Powell, Cleveland, Ohio
- Paul L. Ruflin, Cleveland, Ohio
- David M. Shade, Chicago, Illinois
- Donald J. Thieme, Boston, Massachusetts
- George W. Whetsell, Baltimore, Maryland

A special thank-you to Anne L. Seidensticker, Thomas M. Feuerstein, and Nancy Mravetz. Anne, a health care consultant in our Frankfurt, West Germany office, reviewed, organized, and coordinated the efforts to develop this book. Her help contributed immeasurably to its completeness and comprehensiveness. We hope Anne can implement many of the ideas in the book when she returns to Europe. Tom, a consultant in our National office, reviewed and edited the final drafts of the text. Nancy's patience and direction helped transform written material into a professional and comprehensible form.

In addition to the Ernst & Whinney executives noted above, we appreciate the assistance of our health care clients. Without their real-life experiences, this book would not be possible. We hope their collective efforts will help other health care organizations achieve their cost management objectives.

Finally, the authors would like to thank the editorial staff of Aspen Publishers, Incorporated. Their insights and recommendations were extremely beneficial in ensuring the high quality and clarity of the manuscript.

This publication was prepared for Aspen Publishers, Incorporated, to provide a framework to assist top management, middle management, and students of health care delivery systems to understand the concepts of cost management and their application to the health care industry. Its contents are not based on theory or suppositions. Rather, they reflect a collection of experience, formulated and polished during the design and implementation of numerous cost management systems for health care providers. Anyone planning to develop a cost management system will enhance that undertaking by understanding the concepts and applications presented in this book.

John G. Nackel, Ph.D.
Principal, Ernst & Whinney

# chapter 1

# *Introduction*

## BACKGROUND

Hospitals are faced with an environment of growing competition, changing payment mechanisms, and consolidation. These factors and others challenge hospital boards and management to respond with better management systems, better communication, and better human resource management. Hospitals face growing challenges to maintain or expand their share of a decreasing market by achieving these capabilities. By not responding to the changes, they risk their very survival.

Hospitals also have objectives common to other businesses. For example, they must remain profitable in order to serve their communities effectively and to embrace capital markets for plant and technology modernization. The services they deliver must be of high quality to attract and retain customers in a competitive marketplace. Finally, they have significant human resource and management systems issues to address.

Given these changes, it is more critical than ever for hospitals to examine their environment—today and projected into the future—and to plan courses of action to ensure their survival. For some hospitals, the competitive marketplace has caused major problems. Their ability to react has been severely constrained by antiquated management structures and information systems. This has forced them into a position of reaction instead of proaction—making it difficult for them to improve their market, operational, or financial position. However, a growing number of hospitals are taking aggressive and innovative postures in the health care marketplace. These hospitals are developing effective management and information structures to secure their positions, today and tomorrow.

A key feature of these new management and information structures is an enhanced ability to manage hospital costs. Before the Medicare Prospective Payment System (PPS) and the influx of fixed-price payment schemes, hospitals were more concerned with increasing revenues. Since many insurers paid published charges and Medicare reimbursed hospitals based on costs, the cost of operations was of secondary concern. However, in order to retain or increase their profitability levels today, providers need to focus on the cost of operations to manage their profitability more effectively. A closer analysis of the two components of profitability—revenue and cost of operations—makes this conclusion even more obvious.

## Revenue

With insurers and employers pressuring hospitals for discounts on fees, profit margins are expected to shrink. Similarly, with pressures to reduce or prevent hospital stays in favor of "less costly" alternative treatment modes—for example, home care, ambulatory surgery centers, and birthing centers—inpatient revenues are expected to shrink. These factors are influencing hospitals to pursue new ways, other than traditional rate increases, to maintain or improve profitability levels.

## Cost of Operations

For many hospitals, in order to maintain or improve profit levels, the ability to manage, control, and reduce costs has become a viable alternative to increasing rates. In an atmosphere of competition, changing payment mechanisms, and consolidation, costs have a dramatic impact on many decisions facing hospital management. Costs of services also influence revenue to the extent that they influence pricing decisions. The goal is to reduce operating costs, to increase productivity and profitability, and to become more price competitive.

Applications of cost information include the ability to analyze and improve the profitability of the patient types (for example, DRGs) and product lines (for example, cardiology services). This application helps the provider to expand market share—and profitability—selectively by aggressively seeking out contractual arrangements with health maintenance organizations (HMOs) or preferred provider organizations (PPOs), or by pursuing geographic areas for those products demonstrating high profitability and potential demand.

Another application of cost information is to provide patient treatment information to physicians. This information helps physicians initiate more consistent and effective treatment protocols. Additionally, treatment information may serve as a means to evaluate the effectiveness and economics of alternative treatment regimens and technologies. The net effect of this application is to reduce costs, increase profitability, and improve the quality of care.

A key feature of a cost management information system is flexibility in developing solutions to address the hospital's most pressing issues. A cost management system accomplishes this by recognizing that clinical, financial, and operational issues are interrelated and by providing information that reflects the impact that changes in one issue have on the others. In this way, strategic and management decisions are made with increased confidence, consistency, and accountability—helping all levels of management to perform more effectively and efficiently.

## Cost Information Benefits

What benefits does better cost information provide to managers and clinicians? The answer to this question relates to the particular questions the managers and clinicians address, their responsibilities and authority, and their personal and professional environments.

Top management and the governing body address strategic issues as well as operational issues. Strategic issues include expanding or divesting product lines; forming joint ventures, acquisitions, and mergers; and entering into contractual arrangements to provide medical care for a specific constituency of patients. Operational issues include determining and monitoring effective and economic staffing levels and securing the raw material and equipment resources required to meet a projected level of demand.

Information that is critical to deal effectively with these issues includes accurate, consistent, and timely cost information. For example, before a decision is made regarding an acquisition, the return on investment (profitability), as well as competition and demand, must be examined. Dynamically linked to strategic decisions are the effects each decision has on the cost of operations, that is, how the costs of production change, based on the strategic decision, and how these costs impact the ability of the organization to deliver a competitive, yet profitable, product that is consistent with the organization's mission and philosophy. Cost information serves as one yardstick to measure and stratify the level of investment and return for products that are competing for a limited amount of resources.

Cost information also augments the income determination and financial reporting process. For example, by properly accounting for a product or a product-line's costs, a measure of profitability and return on investment can be calculated. This information provides vital insights to top management and the board regarding the achievement of the financial aspects of the strategic plan. In addition, it can be helpful in complying with external reporting requirements.

Functional managers (for example, department managers) require accurate, consistent, and timely cost information to plan, monitor, and control effectively the resources for which they are responsible. With such information, they can maximize their ability quickly and effectively to pinpoint areas where improvements in operations are needed to meet both least-unit-cost and quality goals. In addition, cost standards can be used as an independent means of identifying and rewarding outstanding performance.

From a clinical standpoint, physicians require improved cost information to analyze the effect of alternative treatment regimens, both clinically and financially. This, in turn, influences capital purchases and alternative treatment programs at strategic and operational levels. Additionally, the quality and effectiveness of care often improve as a result of correcting operational, delivery, and clinical problems.

Finally, product-line managers need information to market effectively the products they are responsible for managing. This includes cost information to help them construct price schedules in response to HMOs and to market services proactively to a target group of consumers. Product-line managers also need accurate cost information to serve as the basis for determining their managerial performance and the performance of their product lines.

## PURPOSE AND ORGANIZATION OF THE BOOK

### Purpose

The purpose of this book is to provide a framework to help the reader understand the application of cost management to the health care industry. The scope of topics covers fundamental cost management concepts, a practical approach to implement a cost management system successfully, and ways to use cost management information to enhance an institution's management and competitive position. The text provides a sound reference for virtually all levels of management—executives, physicians, board members, and functional and product-line managers—regarding cost management concepts and applications. It also addresses the cost issues health care management students should understand before entering the employment market.

We hope that a close examination of these topics and issues will help the reader to recognize the importance of cost management as one of the key concepts in building a more effective management and in achieving long-term survival.

### Organization

Over the past several years, examples of specific hospital cost management components have appeared in the literature. Generally absent from the literature, however, has been a clear understanding of what cost management is, what its application to health care delivery systems entails, and what an appropriate cost management structure might be. To provide the reader with the relevant information and structure, this book is organized in three basic parts.

The first part, *Understanding Cost Management*, builds the foundation for understanding cost management and determining how it can add value to an existing information system's capabilities. The initial chapter, Economic Concepts of Cost Management, describes the origin and uses of cost management in other industries, contrasting many of the concepts and uses with their application to health care, and defining key terminology. The second chapter, Overview of a Hospital Cost Management System, conceptually describes the components and functions of hospital cost management systems. The final chapter in this part presents the practical considerations of cost management. It discusses various degrees of applicability of cost management to different types of hospitals—based on demographic factors (for example, urban or rural location) and market factors (for example, competition within the hospital's marketplace).

The second part, *Developing a Cost Management System*, consists of four chapters that progressively address the steps necessary to define and implement a cost management system. These steps provide alternative approaches, where applicable, to allow the maximum amount of flexibility when tailoring them to the reader's unique situation.

Two chapters in the second part, Setting Procedure Standard Cost Profiles and Establishing Product Resource Consumption Profiles, contain technical discussions of ways to develop these two key components of a cost management system. These chapters purposely contain a substantial portion of the text, since it is the realization of these two components that provides the foundation of a cost management system—and subsequently the confidence of and utility to its end users.

The third part, *Applications of Cost Management Information*, discusses the practical applications of cost management information. Specific chapters address the integration of cost management information with the hospital's management practices—involving organizational restructuring, performance evaluation and compensation systems, and strategic business planning. This third part demonstrates how hospitals can build upon a cost management structure to address managerial and market issues effectively, today and in the future.

After completing this book, we hope the reader will have gained a better understanding of the significant benefits cost management can bring to a health care institution. We have tried to cover all aspects of hospital cost management. We strongly recommend that the entire book be read in order to gain a detailed understanding of cost management. However, we also are aware that the interests of readers may differ greatly.

To provide readers with the information most critical to their particular objectives and responsibilities, we have identified the chapters we think are most important to various types of readers. Table 1–1 outlines the chapters we would recommend, keyed to the specific management positions and responsibilities of various readers.

**Table 1–1** Recommended Chapters Based on Management Position

| Chapters | Top Management | Department Managers | Product-Line Managers | Clinicians | Cost Accountants (System Implementers) | Students |
|---|---|---|---|---|---|---|
| Part I—Understanding Cost Management | | | | | | |
| Economic Concepts of Cost Management | | X | X | | X | X |
| Overview of a Hospital Cost Management System | X | X | X | | X | X |
| Practical Considerations of Implementation | X | | | | X | |
| Part II—Developing a Cost Management System | | | | | | |
| Defining the System | | | | | X | |
| Implementing the System | | | | | X | |
| Setting Procedure Standard Cost Profiles | | X | X | X | X | X |
| Establishing Product Resource Consumption Profiles | | X | X | X | X | X |
| Part III—Applications of Cost Management Information | | | | | | |
| Organizational Structures to Achieve Cost Management | X | X | X | X | X | X |
| Managing with Cost Information | X | X | X | X | X | X |
| A Strategic Cost Management Model | X | X | X | X | X | X |

# part I

# UNDERSTANDING COST MANAGEMENT

# chapter 2

# *Economic Concepts of Cost Management*

## INTRODUCTION

Cost management systems for health care evolved from the cost accounting systems developed by manufacturing industries over many decades. They evolved from inventory valuation and income determination systems (cost accounting systems) into systems that provide information for strategic, operational, clinical, and human resource decision making (cost management systems). Thus, cost management systems have become popular and have spread to service industries—including hospitals—because of their sound business value and broad management applications.

This chapter addresses the ways cost information is used by other industries and defines key terminology used throughout the book. By examining the uses of cost information by other industries, their parallels and dissimilarities in applications to health care management can be drawn.

## WHAT IS COST MANAGEMENT?

Cost management is the ongoing process of planning, monitoring, and controlling operations to meet the strategic direction of the organization. It provides a logical and organized approach to balancing profitability, quality, and mission-related objectives.

Cost management information helps plan and control the cost and quality of patient care and to determine competitive, yet profitable, prices. Therefore, cost management is also an encompassing management philosophy, viewing all organizations—including hospitals—as businesses, within the context of their missions and goals.

How does cost management differ from cost accounting? Originally, cost accounting referred to the ways of accumulating and assigning historical costs to units of products and to departments, primarily for purposes of inventory valuation and income determination. Today, the information that a cost accounting system provides goes far beyond that involved in the gathering and assigning of costs. Such information is now used for the management of operations, for strategic decision making, and for the facilitation of operational and organizational procedures. Due to this metamorphosis from an accounting to a management tool, we refer to these new types of information systems as cost management information systems.

## USES OF COST INFORMATION

The gathering, reporting, and analysis of cost information is typically used for:

- inventory valuation and income determination
- product pricing
- strategic and operational planning and control

### Inventory Valuation and Income Determination

Historically, cost accounting systems were developed to value inventory and to help determine income for a reporting period. For manufacturing industries, the proper recognition or matching of costs with revenues is crucial, since a substantial portion of a period's outputs are typically not sold to customers within that same period. Therefore, the costs related to products sold and the costs of products stocked (inventoried) must be separated in order to determine a particular product's cost and the company's income. Inventory costs are assets, benefitting future periods, while costs of goods sold are expenses, costs that resulted in revenue recognition and that benefitted the current period. This separation process helps determine income for internal and external financial reporting requirements.

The valuation of inventory takes place at several levels of detail. For example, during a particular period's production cycle, the number of cars (finished products) produced by an automobile manufacturer may not equal demand. The costs of the components required to build each car—engine, doors, tires, assembly time, and so on—are determined and assigned to each completed car. The mechanism used to document and describe these components is a bill of materials. The bill of materials provides the definition of the product and lists the type, quantity, and cost of the individual components required to produce a unit of the finished product. An abbreviated example of a bill of materials for a car is presented in Exhibit 2–1.

**Exhibit 2–1**  An Example of a Bill of Materials

Sleek Sports Car—Z Model
Description: 2 Doors
         6-Cylinder Engine
         5-Speed Standard Transmission
         Power Steering
         Power Brakes
         Z-Series Options

| Component | Unit Quantity | Unit Cost | Extended Cost |
|---|---|---|---|
| Fender—Front | 2 | $45.30 | $90.60 |
| Tire—Radial | 4 | 35.22 | 140.88 |
| Assembly Labor— | | | |
|    Front Fender | 2 | 6.41 | 12.82 |
| Assembly Labor—Tire | 4 | 3.63 | 14.52 |
| . | . | . | . |
| . | . | . | . |

For inventory valuation, the count of cars, by type and options, sold and stocked from the period's production is determined. Next, the costs of each are determined and reported either as inventory cost or as cost of goods sold.

Other levels of inventory valuation—for example, for subassemblies and raw materials—typically take place in manufacturing industries. Subassemblies are components of a finished product that require fabrication or fitting together before they can be used. When building a car, an engine is assembled and bolted onto the chassis. The engine is a separate component of the car, generally manufactured independently of finished product production levels; thus, enough are readily on hand or stocked as replacement parts for existing car owners. As with finished products, the costs of their components—cylinders, assembly labor, and so on—can be tracked and attached to those units sold and to those units inventoried, as parts of a finished car or as replacement parts.

Finer levels of detail, represented by raw materials, also are commonly inventoried by manufacturing companies. For an automobile manufacturer, these items typically include cylinders, spark plugs, fenders, and so on. The cost of these items is the purchase price paid to an outside supplier or to another division within the same organization. Other items, such as office forms, may be too minor in dollar amount to be inventoried and are charged off in the current period as administrative costs.

Is inventory valuation a cost accounting application that can be used by hospitals? The answer is yes. Yet, inventory valuation does not have a significant management application in health care.

As in building a car, the various services (tests and treatments) used to treat a patient are documented over the course of the illness. At the end of a reporting period, the costs of patients discharged (like those of the finished product in manufacturing) and the costs of patients currently undergoing treatment (like those of the in-process inventory in manufacturing) must be segregated to match costs properly with revenues for product costing and income determination purposes. However, a unique problem confronting hospitals is that a standard definition of a finished product does not exist. In manufacturing industries, finished products are generally homogeneous in nature, with the identical, engineered bill of materials being used for a specifically defined product. In hospitals, however, each patient is unique, and the patient classification (the product type in manufacturing) may not be known until discharge. Therefore, standard product definitions and standard bills of materials (for example, treatment protocols) are more difficult for hospitals to establish.

Unlike the process in manufacturing industries, most components that go into a hospital's finished products cannot be inventoried. Hospitals do not have a supply of chest x-rays on hand to be used randomly during the treatment of a patient. Most treatments are unique to an individual patient, since they require the patient to be physically present for treatment. Only a few of the components are nonpatient specific (for example, materials like admission kits and medical devices, such as prostheses) and therefore can be inventoried if they are significant in number and dollar amounts.

Unlike the situation in many manufacturing concerns, labor-related costs are the most significant production costs in a hospital. In defining and controlling costs, the nature and extent of labor costs pose a unique challenge to hospitals. Unlike supplies, labor hours cannot be inventoried and are, therefore, incurred whether or not they are consumed in production. Hospitals are hesitant to expand and contract their labor forces as frequently as manufacturers adjust inventory levels. This results in a tendency to classify all full-time employees as fixed labor, beyond the control of cost management or productivity systems.

Finally, the raw materials (chemicals, films, raw drugs) used to manufacture hospital "subassemblies" are generally inventoried periodically only if the items are significant in dollar amount. Their costs are not attached to any patient at a particular point in time; rather they remain within the cost center that is responsible for their administration, much as they do with the hospital's manufacturing counterpart.

Inventory valuation and income determination were historically the thrust of cost accounting systems. However, by determining the labor, material, and other costs associated with manufacturing each component of the finished product and by determining the time required to assemble the finished product itself, a basis was formed to use cost accounting information as a managerial tool. (The managerial applications of cost accounting—product pricing and strategic and operational planning and control—are examined in a later context.)

## Product Pricing

Determining competitive, yet profitable, prices for products requires a comprehensive knowledge of the products' cost and sales volume. Not only is an awareness of historical costs and sales performance required, but also a knowledge of future costs and sales is needed to formulate a pricing policy that secures the recovery of costs and produces a profit. While supply and demand issues, market considerations, and environmental factors still form the foundation of a sound pricing policy, the proper knowledge and application of costs in pricing decisions cannot be ignored.

Manufacturers rely on cost, market, and competitor data when pricing their products. In addition, their pricing policies must be flexible and timely to respond to promotional competition (for example, rebates), changing markets, or competitive challenges. With a complete knowledge of costs and the factors that influence the costs, uncertain future events can be addressed more effectively to ensure acceptable profit levels.

Hospitals must be prepared to price their products strategically to secure competitive contracts from third-party payers, with alternative delivery organizations, and/or directly with major employers. Further complicating matters for hospitals are the myriad product definitions on which they are asked to base their bids. For example, hospitals have been asked to bid on contracts based on product lines, such as all cardiology services, on surgical procedure, such as balloon angioplasty, or on other attributes, such as patient days. In these circumstances, hospitals' tools and policies to assist in pricing decisions must have sufficient flexibility to permit the evaluation of alternative scenarios in a timely manner.

## Strategic and Operational Product Planning and Control

In manufacturing, as in other industries, product planning is generally performed at two levels: the strategic level and the operational level. At both levels, the use of cost information for product planning changes a cost accounting system from an historical accounting tool to a managerial tool.

### Strategic Product Planning

Strategic product planning is the process of determining which products or product lines the organization should offer its customers, and in which markets. In conjunction with these decisions, the organization must determine how the products or product lines will be manufactured and delivered. In determining what products will be manufactured, what the level of production will be, and how the products will be manufactured, it becomes apparent that strategic and operational product planning are dynamically linked.

Strategic product planning for manufacturers involves top management, product-line managers, and plant managers. The necessity of combining the expertise and inputs of all these groups in the strategic product planning process reflects the interdependencies that strategic decisions have on all aspects of the organization.

The various relevant groups must collectively analyze potential demand, competition, return on investment (net revenue over cost), capitalization requirements, and historical performance. Available capacity, suppliers, subcontractors, and overall personnel requirements also must be examined to determine the ability to deliver the finished products on time, at anticipated costs, and at an appropriate level of quality. Capital requirements for new technologies or plant expansion/ modernization must be analyzed to determine their effect on current reserves or to show which financing option is most attractive. Quality considerations are also an integral part of both the strategic and the operational product plan. Even though cost targets per unit of output are reached, it is of little consequence if the finished product is of low quality. Low quality will generally cause sales to suffer, ultimately affecting the attainment of the strategic product plan objectives.

All of these issues need to be addressed for existing product lines and when determining the feasibility of launching new products or product lines. The finalization of the components sets the strategic tone, objectives, and targets of the entire organization.

Strategic product planning for the hospital is similar in process and participation to that of the hospital's manufacturing counterpart. Board members, top management, and physicians review key criteria and set the strategic plan that determines the overall goals and objectives of the hospital for the upcoming fiscal period and beyond.

One of the critical problems confronting hospitals during the strategic product planning process has been the limited availability of product demand information—due to the lack of product definition homogeneity and unreliable product identification processing (for example, inconsistent ICD-9-CM coding). Another major problem for hospitals is that demand is influenced by many external factors, making demand generally sporadic and unpredictable in nature, in contrast with the demand factor for manufacturers who set production levels. Still another compounding factor has been the absence of reporting on the actual performance of products and product lines compared with expectations and targets, as a basis for determining where to invest or divest resources.

These issues were of relatively minor concern when most hospital revenues were based on retrospectively determined costs and fees-for-service at published charges. However, with fixed payment and capitation systems, accurate forecasting of demand and profitability, in conjunction with the monitoring of actual performance against expectations, is crucial to future strategic decision making and the organization's viability. In addition, the determination of sound and consistent profitability and utilization levels is required to embrace capital markets successfully.

One of the reasons that strategic planning in hospitals has been neglected is that there has been an almost unlimited ability to subsidize losses on specific services. Losses within a service area could be subsidized by cost-based reimbursement payments or by increasing charges for fee-for-service payers. Now, the advent of fixed payment and competitive pricing payment mechanisms has banished the idea that "more (of everything) is better." Strategic planning now has gained a new priority and has created new information needs.

### Operational Planning

Operational planning is the construction of a program to deliver (manufacture) the types and quantities of products forecasted for each production cycle. In most organizations, this translates into labor, material, and equipment resources. It requires that decisions be made regarding those areas of manufacturing that will be subcontracted— based on a combination of cost, timing, and quality considerations— and regarding the coordination of work flows between departments to ensure the availability of subassemblies.

Hospitals are similar to other industries when it comes to planning operations. They use forecasts of departmental activity to plan staffing and other resource requirements. For many hospitals, however, departmental activity forecasts generally have been formulated independently of product forecasts, and at a total activity level (for example, total x-ray procedures). This has been due mainly to management philosophy and the lack of software systems to accumulate and process required data. Often, however, it has resulted in significant differences between planned activity forecasts and actual activity levels, causing significant disparities between forecasted costs and actual costs incurred.

Further complicating matters for hospitals is the fact that the demand for each department—number of patients, required tests, or treatments—on any given day and the timing and scheduling of procedures and exams are difficult to anticipate. This is primarily due to emergency cases, patients' conditions and their responses to treatments, varying durations of treatment (for example, surgical procedures), and the absence of a standard assembly process (the type, order, and number of procedures performed for a patient) that is used by all physicians. Unlike manufacturing industries, hospitals cannot take excess operational production (for example, the number of x-ray procedures) on a given day and stockpile (inventory) outputs for subsequent use, because of the uniqueness of the diagnostics and treatments for each patient.

Management exercises control by periodically comparing actual performance with preestablished plans and targets. Historical information—actual costs and activity—are compared with future-oriented information (plans and budgets) to make decisions relating to the present. Information from the past is used to augment current and future decisions and to monitor the degree to which planned objectives are accomplished. These comparisons produce a series of performance reports. Management interprets the results of these reports to determine the magnitude and cause of unexpected performance results. This is management by exception, the concentration of efforts on those areas reporting significant problems and ignoring areas that are basically problem-free. Corrective actions are initiated to control problem areas and to bring costs back into line with expectations.

For management control to work successfully in any organization, several fundamental rules must be followed. First, to be effective, management control must take place at both strategic and operational levels simultaneously. This reflects the interdependencies of performance deviations at the two levels.

Second, responsibility must be defined during the planning phase. This leads to a clear understanding of both expectations and authority on a consistent basis. Responsibility must be limited to those elements that the individual can control; a thorough analysis of the sales and production process is generally required to determine which specific elements each manager can actually control.

Third, the accountability for patient volume must be ensured. Most hospital product sales' forecasts are based on physicians' input. Yet, though physicians do admit the patients, they generally do not admit them to only one hospital. Therefore, since the "sales force" is not working for the company, accountability for patient volumes is severely limited. As more hospitals organize on a product-line basis and more physicians become hospital-based, the accountability for and the accuracy of product and product-line volume forecasts should increase.

Finally, the financial performance of the hospital's products must be monitored accurately. In the past, the monitoring of the profitability of products and product lines has been difficult, since their costs were not known. Historically, their costs were either based on a ratio of costs to charges (RCC) or they were just never entered into the decision-making process. Given the subjectivity and limitations of RCCs, it was arguable whether a given product or product line was profitable or not. Because of the limitations or absence of solid cost data, the requisite comparisons, accountabilities, and controls were often lacking in hospitals at strategic (product) levels. A cost management system that incorporates standard costs provides a means to monitor accurately the financial performance of health care products.

## Operational Variance Analysis

The operational plan (budget) becomes the yardstick by which actual performance can be evaluated. During and after a period's production, comparisons should be made between actual and planned resource levels, material unit prices, and other items. Before processing performance reports, responsibility for each component of the operational budget must be assigned to and assumed by specific individuals. In manufacturing companies, the plant managers, division managers, and foremen are generally responsible for the assembly and construction resources for the organization's various outputs. The costs of each resource component (for example, salaries and wages, purchase prices of raw materials, and so on) are generally the responsibility of personnel managers and purchasing agents.

After assigning and accepting responsibility, performance (variance) reports are produced periodically (daily, weekly, monthly, or quarterly), for productivity and efficiency monitoring in each financial reporting cycle, for managerial purposes and for internal and external reporting. Variances provide significant information and insights on both atypical and exemplary behavior. Based on such information, changes can be quickly and efficiently focused on those areas that are exhibiting problems, and excellent performance can be quantified and rewarded.

The types of variances typically reported for manufacturing companies involve the price and quantity of materials and the wage rate and efficiency of labor. Other factory overhead variances—such as spending, idle capacity, and efficiency—reflect the successes and failures in controlling the variable and fixed overhead expenses of each department.

However, information regarding variances is not an end in itself; it serves rather as the focal point for further analysis and investigative actions. The data on variances enable management to ascertain the degree of discrepancies—either positive or negative—and to make adjustments to eliminate undesirable performance and encourage and reward performance in excess of expectations.

As a function of a cost management system, operational variance analysis can be applied successfully to hospitals. However, because of the general absence of procedure-level standard costs, most hospitals are limited to comparing actual expenditures with planned amounts, resulting in a total variance. While some knowledge of performance is better than none, it is nearly impossible to determine the cause of a total variance, to assign accountability to the responsible individuals, and to initiate corrective actions quickly and effectively. In the future, as more hospitals develop standard costs and analyze their production processes, variance analysis will provide them with the same benefits that other industries have received from their cost management systems—greater control and accountability, cost reductions, increased productivity, and better use of the organization's assets.

## DEFINITIONS OF KEY TERMS

To address the broad needs of various disciplines using a cost management system, definitions of key terms should be standardized. While no definition will erase all doubt about its meaning, it is necessary to provide a framework that facilitates a consistent understanding of key terms by all managers in the organization.

The term *cost* has been defined by various authoritative accounting organizations and noted academicians. In one accounting research study, cost is defined as "an exchange price, a foregoing, a sacrifice made to ensure benefit. In financial accounting, the foregoing or sacrifice at date of acquisition is represented by a current or future diminution in cash or other assets" (Sprouse and Moonitz 1962, 25). The Committee on Cost Concepts and Standards of the American Accounting Association has defined cost as "a foregoing, measured in monetary terms, incurred or potentially to be incurred to achieve a specific objective" (Report of the Committee on Cost Concepts and Standards 1952, 176).

Often, "cost" is used synonymously with "expense." *Expense* is best defined as an expired cost. Expenses measure the amount of decreases in assets or increases in liabilities related to the production and delivery of goods and services. Therefore, expenses are matched with the revenue generated during the reporting period. Costs may be recognized as expenses or as assets having utility for future periods.

Cost can have a series of descriptors that qualify its meaning for a specific purpose. Each descriptor helps explain how the cost is used in direct relation to a specific application. Some of the most common of these descriptors are direct, indirect, fixed, variable, standard, product, overhead, past, and future. Further explanations of these and other cost descriptors will be presented as our discussion of a cost management system proceeds.

Many of the cost terms mentioned are used to describe cost accumulation activities for inventory costing and product pricing, to prepare periodic financial statements, and to plan and control the activities and costs that are the responsibilities of the organization's various levels of management. At times, it is useful to discuss each term in relation to the purpose it serves, since each term is not intended to serve all purposes to the same degree.

## TYPES OF COST

To facilitate the reader's understanding of the application and importance of cost management, our discussion of cost, and its various descriptors, may be organized in four components:

1. cost information in relation to time frames
2. costs that change in relation to volume or time
3. cost data utilized for product pricing
4. costs relating to strategic and operational planning and control

The four types of costs may tend to overlap at times. This is due to the interrelationships of the cost data that are required by a cost management system to fulfill its various functions.

### Cost Information in Relation to Time Frames

A cost management system processes information associated with past, present, and future events. Inventory valuation and the periodic reporting of financial performance mainly utilize information relating to the past. The monitoring and control of sales and operations relate to the present. Planning (budgeting) and analyzing information relate to events that are oriented toward the future. Yet, each aspect of cost information—whether it is oriented to the past, present, or future—is related to other aspects: past performance is used to formulate future plans, and historical costs are used to monitor and control the achievement of planned objectives.

Historical cost information is important, since performance must be reported internally to managerial levels and externally to governmental and regulatory organizations and to owners. However, future cost and profitability information is also critical to the success of any organization. Any changes made in the organization's strategic and/or operating position will affect future periods. The past can be referenced, but not changed.

The success of a cost management system and a cost management philosophy depends on more than accounting for historical information. A proper blend and balancing of information to respond to past, present, and future events are critical to the effective use of a cost management system.

### Costs that Change in Relation to Volume or Time

The total amount of some costs change in direct proportion to increases or decreases in production volume; these are variable costs. Conversely, other costs are static in amount, regardless of production volume, generally changing evenly or intermittently over time; these are fixed costs. On a per-unit basis, variable costs remain static in amount, while fixed costs fluctuate, depending on the level of activity. A cost management system must recognize this distinction if it is to be used effectively for costing and pricing individual products and for developing strategic and operational plans.

Variable costs typically exhibit these qualities:

- The total amount of the costs fluctuate in direct proportion to changes in volume.
- The cost per unit of output generally remains constant.
- The costs are ratably consumed during the production process.
- The costs are the responsibility of the managerial level in charge of the production process.

Graphically, the behavior of variable costs on a per-unit-of-output basis and in total amount, in relation to volume, may be shown as in Figure 2–1.

The qualities exhibited by fixed costs include the following:

- The total amount of the fixed costs remains constant regardless of changes in volume.
- As volume increases or decreases, the fixed cost per unit decreases or increases correspondingly.

The behavior of fixed costs on a per-unit basis and in total amount, as they relate to changes in volume, is graphically displayed in Figure 2–2.

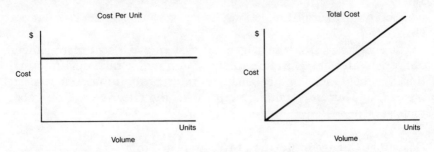

**Figure 2–1**  Variable Cost Behavior

The capabilities of cost management and transaction systems (for example, general ledger) generally preclude categorizing costs other than as fixed or variable. However, sometimes costs are semifixed or semivariable in nature, possessing both fixed and variable components within a relevant range of activity. A graphic illustration of semifixed/variable cost behavior is presented in Figure 2–3.

While semivariable costs change based on relevant range production levels, costs previously categorized as fixed or variable also may be affected by relevant range issues, thus placing them in different categories.

The relevant range is the corridor of activity in which costs categorized as fixed and variable generally behave according to those categorizations. However, certain costs may behave differently if the activity extends beyond the parameters of the relevant range. For example, if a diagnostic radiology department's activity continually decreases, its personnel may have to be laid off, and the supervisory personnel who previously performed strictly supervisory (fixed) activities may be reassigned to perform both supervisory and production (variable) activities. Due to the dynamics of demand in most markets, it is critical to document the activity points where cost behavior changes. By under-

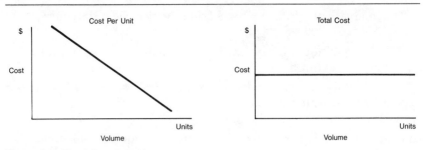

**Figure 2–2**  Fixed-Cost Behavior

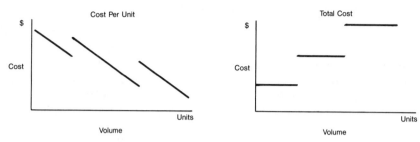

**Figure 2–3** Semifixed/Variable Cost Behavior

standing how and when costs change according to changes in levels of activity, organizations can improve their budgeting and control.

### Cost Data Utilized for Product Pricing

In most organizations, the cost of products has production labor, materials, and equipment components. These components can be further subdivided into direct and indirect categories. In addition, institutional overhead costs must be identified and logically assigned to products to determine the full cost of each unit of output.

Direct production cost components are those items that are specifically traceable to the production of a unit of output. The organization must be able to measure the amount of each cost component expended during the production process. Generic examples of direct production labor activities are assembly, packaging, and processing. Examples of direct production materials are steel, fabric, and plastics for a manufacturer, and x-ray film, developer, and film jackets for a hospital. Examples of direct production equipment resources are baking ovens, welders, and riveters for a manufacturer, and radiology equipment, blood analyzers, and lithotripters for a hospital.

Indirect production cost components encompass those labor, material, and equipment costs that do not specifically contribute to the production of an individual unit of output. Rather, they exist for the operation and convenience of the production process as a whole. Also included in this category are those items that are minuscule in cost or that are incidental to the production process. Examples of generic indirect labor activities are supervision time, the preparation of management reports, and the ordering of supplies. Examples of indirect materials are cleaning agents, staples/tacks, and interoffice communication forms. Examples of indirect equipment are chairs, cabinets, and storage bins.

Both direct and indirect production cost components can be segregated into fixed and variable categories (based on the criteria previously discussed). For example, the charting of a patient's record is an indirect variable labor function. The total amount of indirect time spent by nursing personnel on this function varies in proportion to the number and type of patients on the nursing unit. Recognition of this concept can help to formulate pricing policies and to determine a product's contribution to fixed costs and overhead. Typically, direct production costs are variable, whereas indirect production costs are fixed (discretionary). This distinction is maintained in the budgeting and performance reporting applications of a cost management system. However, there are exceptions, such as equipment, to this rule-of-thumb distinction.

Institutional overhead comprises the costs of those departments that provide support and business services to the organization as a whole. The costs of these departments are allocated to user departments, based on statistics that accurately reflect consumption. Examples of institutional overhead are personnel/payroll functions, switchboard, and marketing. Overhead costs are typically fixed (discretionary) in nature across a broad relevant range.

By using the direct and indirect, fixed and variable, and overhead cost components of each product, individually and in combination, a solid basis on which to establish prices and pricing policies is formed. For example, prices may be based on direct costs, plus a mark-up of a certain percentage or fixed dollar amount per unit; they may be based on a percentage of fully absorbed costs (including all direct, indirect, and overhead costs); or they may be based on variable costs only, plus a mark-up. When coupled with supply and demand projections , product cost information can be used in strategic planning to determine the overall profitability of products and product lines and the collective profitability of the organization as a whole. This, in turn, drives decisions regarding other strategic issues, such as plant modernization, expansion, and acquisitions of other organizations.

### Costs Relating to Strategic and Operational Planning and Control

Two types of costs—budgeted and standard—are integral to strategic and operational planning and control.

Budgeted costs are the costs that are expected to be incurred for future periods, given a forecasted level of the types and volumes of output. Budgeted amounts are determined for direct and indirect production requirements and for institutional overhead. When all aspects of the budgeting process are brought together—sales forecast, production requirements, and administrative costs—the final budget represents the organization's plan for the future period (usually one year).

Standard costs are integrally linked with budgeted costs. Standard costs are based on the types and quantities of resources required to produce a unit of output under normal circumstances, multiplied by each resource's respective unit cost. Standard resources are generally derived through a combination of special studies (for example, time and motion studies) and observations (for example, observation of the production process to identify the method of production). Standard unit costs are determined by reviewing such documents as employment contracts for labor and materials management/purchase contracts for materials. Standard overhead and equipment costs must be viewed in relation to the total production volume forecasted, based on a calculation of the respective costs per unit. Since overhead and equipment costs are fixed in amount, they are rationally spread over the entire volume of output when determining unit costs. For example, if standard (forecasted) equipment and overhead costs total $5,000, and the total volume of output forecasted is 1,000 units, each unit of output will have a standard unit overhead and equipment cost of $5 ($5,000 divided by 1,000 total units to be produced).

Variable unit cost standards are used for both planning and control purposes. For example, they are used for budgeting (planning) the variable portion of the organization's operating budget. This is accomplished by extending variable unit cost standards by forecasted production volumes. The control component uses standards as the benchmark against which actual experience can be evaluated. This standard-to-actual comparative process produces a series of variances that management analyzes to pinpoint variance causes. Using variance analysis, solutions to problems can be more closely focused and are generally more effective. Thus, variance analysis is more a managerial than an accounting function.

Standards may also be used to augment pricing schedules and policies. Standard costs per unit of finished product inform top management of margins and profitability and show how the organization compares with competitors. Decisions based on such information may also impact operational budgets, for example, in cutting back production.

## SUMMARY

The discussion in this chapter has outlined the generic functions and key terminology of a cost management system. As the information needs of organizations change due to internal and external environmental factors, the need for additional and improved information grows. For many organizations, the cost management system effectively provides the requisite information.

By understanding the benefits that cost management has brought to other industries, hospital managers should feel more comfortable in the application of cost management principles to their own organizations. In the remainder of this book, we examine the various tools needed to design, implement, and manage a cost management system.

**REFERENCES**

"Report of the Committee on Cost Concepts and Standards," *Accounting Review* 27(1952).

Robert T. Sprouse and Maurice Moonitz, *A Tentative Set of Broad Accounting Principles for Business Enterprises*, Accounting Research Study No. 3 (New York: American Institute of Certified Public Accountants, 1962).

# chapter 3

# Overview of a Hospital Cost Management System

## INTRODUCTION

In the health care industry, hospital managers use different definitions, and have various understandings of the purpose, of a cost management system. Depending on whom you ask—chief executive officer, chief financial officer, physician, department manager, or product-line manager—each will have a unique, personal understanding of its functions, scope, complexity, and comprehensiveness. However, it is imperative that a consensus on these matters be achieved among the various managerial disciplines, since cost management influences the strategic, financial, clinical, and operational issues addressed by all levels of management. To this end, the discussion in this chapter provides a framework for developing a consistent understanding of hospital cost management issues among readers—and among the end users of the system.

## SYSTEM COMPONENTS

For hospitals, the objective of a cost management system is to provide cost information for strategic market positioning and for the planning, monitoring, and controlling of functional and clinical operations. To accomplish strategic market positioning objectives, a cost management system calculates the costs—both fixed and variable—of products (such as diagnosis related groups—DRGs) in response to competitive bidding requests or for market expansion/selection planning. To plan, monitor, and control functional and clinical operations, a cost management system constructs operational budgets and treatment expectations, and then, through a series of performance reports, monitors actual performance compared with those expectations.

To accomplish these objectives, five logical functions must be performed by a cost management system. Each of these functions may be given greater or lesser emphasis in a specific hospital, based on its unique needs. However, all five functions are generally necessary to achieve the long-term market and management positioning required by most hospitals. The five functions are:

1. *Cost determination*—Profiling the fixed and variable cost components of products (for example, DRGs) and procedures (for example, chest x-rays).
2. *Activity forecasting*—Projecting demand for specific products or product lines (for example, cardiology services) for a particular period of time. The product demand forecast may subsequently be used, based on individual procedures, to drive each hospital cost center's workload demand.
3. *Functional cost center budgeting*—Translating the forecasted workload demand of each cost center into a forecast of labor, supply, and general ledger expense requirements to meet the forecasted demand.
4. *Performance reporting on a product level*—Comparing actual mix and volumes of products with forecasted levels, and comparing actual with expected procedure usage in treating patients within a product line.
5. *Performance reporting on a functional level*—Comparing actual resources and costs incurred with both the planned (for example,

annual) budget plan and with an earned budget (standard resource and cost requirements extended at actual activity).

The sources of cost management data and the logical flow and interrelationships of a cost management system's functions are graphically presented in Figure 3–1.

In the remainder of this chapter, we discuss the objectives, inputs and outputs, and uses of each of these functions of a hospital cost management system.

## Cost Determination

Cost determination (or cost construction) is the profiling of standard costs at two (or more) levels of detail. Most hospitals confine their cost management systems to two levels of detail, in contrast with other industries that may cost individual component parts at finer levels of detail. Hospitals do not define additional levels because of the lack of homogeneity of product definitions, and because of the unacceptable cost/benefit ratio in implementing the data collection systems required to accumulate actual costs at finer levels of detail.

The two levels of standards are defined as *procedural,* the most detailed level of cost, and *product,* representing an aggregation of procedures.

### Procedure Cost Standards

Procedures are discrete services—either clinical or support—provided to patients or other hospital cost centers. In nursing cost centers, they

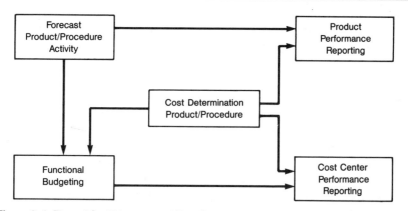

**Figure 3–1** Flow of Cost Management Functions

are typically defined as a day of nursing care at a specified acuity level. In ancillary cost centers, they are generally defined as diagnostic tests or therapeutic treatments performed for a patient. In support cost centers—such as dietary, admitting, and medical records—they are generally not defined as direct patient care. Examples of support cost center procedures are a patient's salt-free diet, admission procedure, and medical record processing. Even cost centers that have been traditionally viewed as overhead can define procedures (activities or outputs) for cost determination and other applications. For example, the resources and costs of a maintenance cost center can be related to the number and magnitude of work orders.

The objective of the cost determination function is to relate hospital costs to specific cost behavior. Cost behavior is the recognition of changes in costs in relation to different levels and types of activity.

For example, hospitals have traditionally incorporated the procedures of multiple patient care and support cost centers (for example, nursing, dietary, admitting) into a single day rate. However, these activities have quite different cost implications for hospitals, since all of them do not, in fact, vary incrementally with a day of stay. Therefore, hospitals need to unbundle their patient care and support costs in the following incremental activity measures:

- *Nursing care.* These costs vary by specific patient. However, since it is difficult to track actual nursing care hours by patient, most hospital cost management systems make use of patient acuity (classification) systems as surrogates for patient-specific cost collection. Thus, an example of a procedure for nursing would be a day of stay at a particular patient acuity level.

- *Day-of-stay costs (hotel services).* These costs vary with each day spent in a specific nursing unit. They include such activities as room and board, laundry, housekeeping, and dietary. Thus, an example of a procedure for day-of-stay costs would be a patient meal.

- *Admission/discharge costs.* These costs vary with a single episode of illness. They represent similar one-time costs for patients who may stay 1 day or 20 days. Typical cost center costs involve admitting, billing, and medical records. Thus, an example of a procedure for admission/discharge costs would be a normal admission; another might be an emergency admission.

- *Diagnostic testing or therapeutic treatment costs.* These costs typically vary by the type and number of tests or treatments and are generally already being captured in the hospital's billing system. An example of a procedure for a diagnostic test would be a complete blood count (CBC) or a chest x-ray.

Any patient care or support service that varies with respect to one of the above activities could be defined as a procedure. However, while many procedures are represented by charge items in the hospital's billing system, others are not. In fact, most hospitals have never had a reason for collecting procedure costs based on cost behavior. The goal of relating cost determination to cost behavior is to recognize and track *incremental* levels of service provided to patients.

For overhead cost centers, procedure activity and cost behavior are measured independently of fluctuations in patient activity. Their calculation is usually based on the number and type of outputs or activities provided to other cost centers or employees. Examples of overhead cost center procedures are maintenance cost center work orders of various duration and the number and duration of visits to the employee health center.

For any defined procedure, a procedure standard resource and cost profile can be developed. Typically, hospitals have utilized ratios of costs to charges (RCCs) or relative value units (RVUs) to estimate the cost of procedures. While RCCs have some value, they are extremely unreliable and inaccurate for most management purposes. RVUs represent a significant improvement in accuracy and may be validly used to allocate total costs to individual procedures. However, they are not reliable for cost monitoring, budgeting, and control. Clearly, the most accurate and reliable costing technique is the procedure standard cost profile. Table 3–1 presents a grid comparing the features and functions of the three costing methodologies.

The procedure standard cost profile identifies the required resources and costs to produce a procedure at a specified level of volume. The detail level may vary. It may be a single figure, recognizing direct labor versus labor requirements by job code, or all supplies versus supplies by general ledger subaccount; but, in any case, it should generally include the following components:

- direct variable costs—labor required to perform the procedure and supplies consumed by the procedure
- indirect variable costs—labor and supply items that fluctuate in proportion with activity, yet are not "hands on" in nature—for example, patient charting, the scheduling of tests, and the prepara-

**Table 3–1** Comparison of Costing Methodologies

| Attribute | Ratio of Cost to Charges | Relative Value Units | Detailed Procedural Costing |
|---|---|---|---|
| Is usually available historically | Y | N | N |
| Has relatively low cost | Y | Y | N |
| Has short time frame to implement | Y | Y | N |
| Is readily available for major departments | Y | Y | N |
| Is supported by existing systems | Y | Y | N |
| Can provide a measure of productivity | N | Y | Y |
| Recognizes fixed and variable cost relationships | N | Y | Y |
| Projects staffing requirements | N | Y | Y |
| Supports flexible budgeting scenarios | N | Y | Y |
| Supports strategic pricing decisions | N | Y | Y |
| Has high degree of maintenance | N | Y | Y |
| Accommodates noncharged patient procedures | N | Y | Y |
| Accommodates overhead departments | N | Y | Y |
| Produces detailed departmental expense budgets | N | N | Y |
| Has high degree of accuracy | N | N | Y |

tion of charge slips—that may or may not be allocated to the procedure

- indirect fixed cost center costs—supervisory salaries, office supplies, and equipment depreciation that are allocated to the procedure
- hospital overhead—building depreciation and interest, data processing, and general management items that are allocated as general business costs.

An example of a typical procedure standard cost profile for a nursing procedure is presented as Exhibit 3–1.

*Product Cost Standards*

In our approach to hospital cost management, a product is defined as an episode of patient care. Products may be separately defined as inpatient products (discharges) and outpatient products (visits), or they may be combined when outpatient preadmission testing and/or aftercare are provided in addition to an inpatient stay.

**Exhibit 3–1** Example of a Procedure Standard Cost Profile

Procedure Standard Resource and Cost Profile

Cost Center: Medical Units
Procedure Name: Nursing Care, Level 4
Procedure No.: 300423

| Production Component | Standard Procedure Usage | | Standard Unit Cost | | Total Standard Cost |
|---|---|---|---|---|---|
| Labor: | | | | | |
| Direct (variable) | | | | | |
| Head nurse | 0.0 Hrs. | × | $14.50 | = | $ .00 |
| RN | 4.9 Hrs. | × | 9.05 | = | 44.35 |
| Aide | 1.6 Hrs. | × | 5.30 | = | 8.48 |
| Unit clerk | 0.2 Hrs. | × | 6.10 | = | 1.22 |
| Indirect (variable) | | | | | |
| Head nurse | 0.1 Hrs. | × | 14.50 | = | 1.45 |
| RN | 0.8 Hrs. | × | 9.05 | = | 7.24 |
| Aide | 0.4 Hrs. | × | 5.30 | = | 2.12 |
| Unit clerk | 0.2 Hrs. | × | 6.10 | = | 1.22 |
| Indirect (fixed) | | | | | |
| Head nurse | 0.3 Hrs. | × | 14.50 | = | 4.35 |
| RN | 0.1 Hrs. | × | 9.05 | = | 0.91 |
| Aide | 0.1 Hrs. | × | 5.30 | = | 0.53 |
| Unit clerk | 0.1 Hrs. | × | 6.10 | = | 0.61 |
| Vacation, holiday, sickness | 0.4 Hrs. | × | 8.65 | = | 3.46 |
| Subtotal | | | | | 75.94 |
| Material: | | | | | |
| Direct (variable) | | | | | |
| Miscellaneous | 1/Day | × | 1.42 | = | 1.42 |
| Indirect (variable) | | | | | |
| Charting supplies | 3/Day | × | 0.26 | = | 0.78 |
| Miscellaneous | 1/Day | × | 0.11 | = | 0.11 |
| Indirect (fixed) | | | | | |
| Office supplies | 1/Day | × | 0.17 | = | 0.17 |
| Subtotal | | | | | 2.48 |
| Cost center overhead: | | | | | |
| Equipment | 1/Day | × | 0.22 | = | 0.22 |
| Other | 1/Day | × | 0.03 | = | 0.03 |
| Subtotal | | | | | .25 |
| Allocated overhead: | | | | | |
| Business functions | 1/Day | × | 22.68 | = | 22.68 |
| Environmental | 1/Day | × | 9.79 | = | 9.79 |
| Research and education | 1/Day | × | 4.25 | = | 4.25 |
| Subtotal | | | | | 36.72 |
| Total procedure cost | | | | | $ 115.39 |

A discharge or a visit is an episode that is too broad to use as a definition for a hospital product. As a result of the Medicare Prospective Payment System (PPS), DRGs have now gained wide acceptance as an appropriate definition. However, DRGs do not address outpatient care, and they are often challenged as nonhomogenous clinical groupings. Disease-stage categories, severity-of-illness categories, and patient management categories are examples of alternative inpatient product measures. Ambulatory visit groupings (AVGs) are an example of an outpatient product measure.

Typically, hospitals use different product definitions simultaneously for different management applications—DRGs for reimbursement analysis, DRGs with severity measures for physician analysis, and strategic program units (SPUs) for planning purposes. Each product definition has specific attributes and a level of detail best suited for its intended use. However, an essential feature of a hospital cost management system is that it must be able to "roll up" flexibly or to summarize procedure costs in different product definitions, depending on the use for which the product profiles are being developed.

Once a product definition is determined, a product resource consumption profile, or bill of materials, should be developed. In the past, many hospitals generated these profiles at the total hospital or cost center level of detail, based on patient charges. Yet, though these aggregate measures may be valid for some analyses, they are quite inadequate for pricing products, strategic planning, and monitoring clinical practices. By our definition, a product resource consumption profile must identify the type and volume of individual procedures that are expected to be consumed in product delivery. The volume of procedures is then costed out, using the procedure standard cost profiles previously described.

An example of a product resource consumption profile is presented as Exhibit 3–2. Note the appearance of the Nursing Care Level 4 procedure and how its standard unit cost can be traced to Exhibit 3–1.

## Activity Forecasting

Activity forecasting takes place at two levels—product and procedure. The first step in the forecasting process is to estimate demand for products. While demand for each product, such as a DRG, may be evaluated, it is generally more meaningful to evaluate the demand for a product line, such as oncology or cardiovascular surgery. Product lines allow a more reasonable analysis of the factors affecting hospital demand, including:

**Exhibit 3–2** Example of a Product Resource Consumption Profile

Product Resource Consumption Profile

Product No.:    DRG No. 139
Product Name: Cardiac Arrhythmia & Conduction Disorders Age < 70 W/O C.C.

| Procedure Number/Name | Standard Procedure Usage | Standard Unit Cost | Total Standard Cost |
|---|---|---|---|
| Admission/discharge procedures | | | |
| 100101  Admission—normal | 1 each  × | $ 26.19  = | $   26.19 |
| 100109  Medical record processing | 1 each  × | 42.12  = | 42.12 |
| 100110  Billing—Medicare | 1 each  × | 19.85  = | 19.85 |
| Nursing procedures | | | |
| 300123  Nursing Care Level 1 | 1 day  × | 43.13  = | 43.13 |
| 300223  Nursing Care Level 2 | 3 days  × | 69.85  = | 209.55 |
| 300323  Nursing Care Level 3 | 4 days  × | 88.42  = | 353.68 |
| 300423  Nursing Care Level 4 | 3 days  × | 115.39  = | 346.17 |
| Day-of-stay procedures | | | |
| 200100  Normal meal | 17 each  × | 8.79  = | 149.43 |
| 200410  Laundry/linen—medical | 9 each  × | 3.38  = | 30.42 |
| 200950  Housekeeping—normal | 11 each  × | 3.13  = | 34.43 |
| Diagnostic and therapeutic procedures | | | |
| 800422  Chest x-ray pa/lat | 1 each  × | 37.39  = | 37.39 |
| 900123  Lab CBC | 1 each  × | 2.85  = | 2.85 |
| 900124  Lab electrolytes | 3 each  × | 16.60  = | 49.80 |
| 700011  EKG—bedside | 1 each  × | 38.99  = | 38.99 |
| 600910  IV therapy | 7 each  × | 22.60  = | 158.20 |
| Total product cost | | | $1,542.20 |

- absolute demand, which is a function of population characteristics, mortality and morbidity rates, product life cycle, synergistic fit with other products (for example, cardiovascular surgery with cardiac rehabilitation programs), and alternative treatment options
- relative demand, which is the hospital's share of the absolute demand, based on competitive factors, medical staff composition, marketing considerations, and the hospital's image and capabilities.

Estimates of these product demands are generally the responsibility of senior hospital management and product-line managers, supplemented by input from key physicians.

Based on historical relationships of individual product (for example, DRG) volumes within a product line, product-line volume forecasts may be spread back to estimate individual product activity. Individual product measures that relate to payments (for example, DRG) are needed to calculate contractual allowances and to prepare cash flow projections.

The product resource consumption profiles constructed in the cost determination process can be used by hospital management to create periodic functional cost center demand forecasts. Traditionally, functional cost center managers, such as the radiology director, have been responsible for forecasting the demand for their procedures. However, radiology procedures are not an independent variable in the forecasting equation; they are dependent variables that are directly related to the volume and type of patients treated.

Once product demand has been forecasted, the volume and type of products that make up the demand forecast (for example, patients to be treated) are extended against their respective resource consumption profiles, producing a forecast of individual procedure activity for each particular product. This extension is performed for all hospital products and then aggregated up to a total inpatient demand, by procedure, for each hospital functional cost center. To complete the procedure activity forecast, outpatient procedure activities—using outpatient product measures, such as AVGs or traditional forecasting techniques—are forecasted and added to each cost center's inpatient procedure activity forecast. This process is depicted in Exhibits 3–3, 3–4, and 3–5.

### Functional Cost Center Budgeting

Given the previously developed forecast of procedure activity, hospital cost center managers are required to plan the production process. Typically, the hospital budget process has relied heavily on historical spending patterns (for example, last year's budget, plus or minus changes in total cost center activity, inflation, and so on). In a cost management system, the forecast of procedure activities is extended by their respective standard resource and cost profiles to develop each cost center's variable expense budget. Fixed expenses and resources are determined by using historical amounts trended forward, on such relationships as required supervision per employee or accreditation requirements. The variable and fixed budget components are added together to arrive at the cost center's total expense and resource budget. Exhibits 3–6 and 3–7 provide examples of this process. While these examples

**Exhibit 3–3** Example of a Procedure Activity Forecast Process

Procedure Activity Forecast Process—One Inpatient Product

Product Resource Consumption Case Profile
DRG No. 139   Cardiac Arrhythmia & Conduction Disorders < 70 W/O C.C.

| Procedure Number/Name | | Standard Procedure Usage | | Forecasted Product Activity | | Procedure Activity Forecast |
|---|---|---|---|---|---|---|
| 100101 | Admission—normal | 1 | × | 650 | = | 650 |
| 100109 | Medical record processing | 1 | × | 650 | = | 650 |
| 100110 | Billing—Medicare | 1 | × | 650 | = | 650 |
| 200100 | Normal meal | 17 | × | 650 | = | 11,050 |
| 200410 | Laundry/linen—medical | 9 | × | 650 | = | 5,850 |
| 200950 | Housekeeping—normal | 11 | × | 650 | = | 7,150 |
| 300123 | Nursing Care Level 1 | 1 | × | 650 | = | 650 |
| 300223 | Nursing Care Level 2 | 3 | × | 650 | = | 1,950 |
| 300323 | Nursing Care Level 3 | 4 | × | 650 | = | 2,600 |
| 300423 | Nursing Care Level 4 | 3 | × | 650 | = | 1,950 |
| 600910 | IV therapy | 7 | × | 650 | = | 4,550 |
| 700011 | EKG—bedside | 1 | × | 650 | = | 650 |
| 800422 | Chest x-ray pa/lat | 1 | × | 650 | = | 650 |
| 900123 | Lab CBC | 1 | × | 650 | = | 650 |
| 900124 | Lab electrolytes | 3 | × | 650 | = | 1,950 |

are oversimplifications, they do illustrate several key concepts in budgeting with procedure standard cost profiles.

The budget for variable costs is driven by the extension of forecasted activities, times standard unit resource requirements and their respective unit costs. The fixed and overhead costs are determined on a cost center basis, generally without regard to individual procedures. Fixed and overhead costs are allocated to procedures to determine the fully absorbed procedure and product costs. These costs can then be used by management for making pricing decisions and for clinical monitoring and control purposes.

The above discussion illustrates the dichotomy inherent in a hospital cost management system. Fully absorbed costs are best suited for product pricing, income determination, and product-line performance monitoring. Variable costs are best suited for cost center budget construction and cost center performance monitoring.

Another factor involved in preparing a budget based on standard resource and cost profiles is planned inefficiency, or the difference

**Exhibit 3–4** Example of an Inpatient Procedure Activity Forecast Process

| | Inpatient Procedure Activity Forecast Process—All Products | | | |
|---|---|---|---|---|
| Procedure Number/Name | 138 Card Arrhyth/Co >69 and/or C.C. | 139 Card Arrhyth/Co <70 W/O C.C. | 140 Angina Pectoris | Totals |
| 300123 Nursing Care Level 1 | 510 + | 650 + | 420 = | 1,580 |
| 300223 Nursing Care Level 2 | 300 + | 1,950 + | 1,900 = | 4,150 |
| 300323 Nursing Care Level 3 | 2,650 + | 2,600 + | 90 = | 5,340 |
| 300423 Nursing Care Level 4 | 2,100 + | 1,950 + | 2,610 = | 6,660 |
| Totals | 5,560 + | 7,150 + | 5,020 = | 17,730 |

between standard and expected staffing plans. Assume that 37,000 RN hours or 18 FTEs (full-time equivalents) are required for the forecasted volume of nursing care. Because of the mix of people in the available labor pool and accreditation requirements, it may not be possible to staff only 18 FTEs, for 100-percent efficiency. For example, the hospital may need to staff five RNs on the night shift, due to the unpredictability of

**Exhibit 3–5** Example of a Cost Center Total Procedure Activity Forecast

| | Cost Center Total Procedure Activity Forecast | | | |
|---|---|---|---|---|
| | | Activity | | |
| Procedure Number/Name | Inpatient | Outpatient | | Total |
| 300123 Nursing Care Level 1 | 1,580 + | 0 | = | 1,580 |
| 300223 Nursing Care Level 2 | 4,150 + | 0 | = | 4,150 |
| 300323 Nursing Care Level 3 | 5,340 + | 0 | = | 5,340 |
| 300423 Nursing Care Level 4 | 6,660 + | 0 | = | 6,660 |
| Totals | 17,730 + | 0 | = | 17,730 |

**Exhibit 3–6** Example of a Cost Forecasting Process for a Single
Procedure

Forecasted Costs—One Procedure

Cost Center:     Medical Units
Procedure Name:     Nursing Care—Level 4
Procedure No.:     300423

| Production Component | Standard Unit Cost | | Forecasted Procedure Volume | | Forecasted Resource Costs |
|---|---|---|---|---|---|
| **Labor:** | | | | | |
| Direct (variable) | | | | | |
| Head nurse | $ — | × | 6,660 | = | $ — |
| RN | 44.35 | × | 6,660 | = | 295,371 |
| Aide | 8.48 | × | 6,660 | = | 56,477 |
| Unit clerk | 1.22 | × | 6,660 | = | 8,125 |
| Indirect (variable) | | | | | |
| Head nurse | 1.45 | × | 6,660 | = | 9,657 |
| RN | 7.24 | × | 6,660 | = | 48,218 |
| Aide | 2.12 | × | 6,660 | = | 14,119 |
| Unit clerk | 1.22 | × | 6,660 | = | 8,125 |
| Indirect (fixed) | | | | | |
| Head nurse | | | | | |
| RN | | | | | |
| Aide | | | | | |
| Unit clerk | | | | | |
| Vacation, holiday, sickness | | | | | |
| Subtotal | 66.08 | | | | 440,092 |
| **Material:** | | | | | |
| Direct (variable) | | | | | |
| Miscellaneous | 1.42 | × | 6,660 | = | 9,457 |
| Indirect (variable) | | | | | |
| Charting supplies | 0.78 | × | 6,660 | = | 5,195 |
| Miscellaneous | 0.11 | × | 6,660 | = | 733 |
| Indirect (fixed) | | | | | |
| Office supplies | | | | | |
| Subtotal | 2.31 | | | | 15,385 |
| **Cost center overhead:** | | | | | |
| Equipment | | | | | |
| Other | | | | | |
| Subtotal | | | | | |
| **Allocated overhead:** | | | | | |
| Business functions | | | | | |
| Environmental | | | | | |
| Research and education | | | | | |
| Subtotal | | | | | |
| **Total procedure** | | | | | |
| Variable costs | $ 68.39 | | | | $455,477 |

**Exhibit 3–7** Example of a Cost Forecasting Process for All Cost Center Procedures

Cost Center:      Medical Units
Procedure Name:   All Procedures
Procedure No.:    N/A

Forecasted Costs—All Cost Center Procedures

| Production Component | 300123 Nursing Care Level 1 | 300223 Nursing Care Level 2 | 300323 Nursing Care Level 3 | 300423 Nursing Care Level 4 | | Total |
|---|---|---|---|---|---|---|
| Labor: | | | | | | |
| Direct (variable) | | | | | | |
| Head nurse | $ — | + $ — | + $ — | + $ — | = | $ — |
| RN | 110,005 | + 145,200 | + 183,708 | + 295,371 | = | 734,284 |
| Aide | 20,332 | + 26,830 | + 34,001 | + 56,477 | = | 137,640 |
| Unit clerk | 1,803 | + 2,400 | + 3,011 | + 8,125 | = | 15,339 |
| Indirect (variable) | | | | | | |
| Head nurse | 3,618 | + 4,777 | + 6,044 | + 9,657 | = | 24,096 |
| RN | 14,820 | + 19,556 | + 24,757 | + 48,218 | = | 107,351 |
| Aide | 4,340 | + 5,726 | + 7,250 | + 14,119 | = | 31,435 |
| Unit clerk | 2,722 | + 3,788 | + 4,545 | + 8,125 | = | 19,180 |
| Indirect (fixed) | | | | | | |
| Head nurse | | | | | | 68,431 |
| RN | | | | | | 13,510 |
| Aide | | | | | | 7,317 |
| Unit clerk | | | | | | 8,096 |
| Vacation, holiday, sickness | | | | | | 62,270 |
| Subtotal | | | | | | 1,228,949 |

| | | | | | | |
|---|---|---|---|---|---|---|
| Material: | | | | | | |
| Direct (variable) | | | | | | |
| Miscellaneous | 3,522 | + | 4,649 | + | 5,881 | + | 9,457 | = | 23,509 |
| Indirect (variable) | | | | | | |
| Charting supplies | 1,935 | + | 2,554 | + | 3,231 | + | 5,195 | = | 12,915 |
| Miscellaneous | 273 | + | 360 | + | 456 | + | 733 | = | 1,822 |
| Indirect (fixed) | | | | | | |
| Office supplies | | | | | | 2,814 |
| Subtotal | | | | | | 41,060 |
| Cost center overhead: | | | | | | |
| Equipment | | | | | | 3,753 |
| Other | | | | | | 496 |
| Subtotal | | | | | | 4,249 |
| Allocated overhead: | | | | | | |
| Business functions | | | | | | 375,490 |
| Environmental | | | | | | 162,082 |
| Research and education | | | | | | 70,363 |
| Subtotal | | | | | | 607,935 |
| Total cost center costs | | | | | | $1,882,193 |

demand or fluctuations in patient nursing (acuity) requirements. There-fore, on this particular unit, the hospital may be forced to staff 20 FTEs, for a 90-percent efficiency rating, despite the standard. Generally, stand-ards should exclude these planned inefficiencies in order to keep targets purely defined, whereas budgets should include them as part of the financial and operating plan in order to forecast realistically what will happen.

**Performance Reporting on a Product Level**

Once a product and procedure forecast is prepared, a hospital can compare actual product activity and treatment regimens with planned levels and resource consumption profiles. A period of case mix data can be compared with the original plan on a DRG, or on another similar product or product-line basis. The results of this comparison will show volume, mix, and treatment variances. Brief explanations of each vari-ance can then be presented. (Further discussion of product variances and their interpretation and use is presented in Part III.)

Volume variances represent the difference between planned and actual individual product activity, using the standard cost per product to quantify the variance. In the example shown in Exhibit 3–3, the hospital expected to produce 650 DRG No. 139 patient discharges. Each patient discharge was planned to average $1,542.20 in cost. If only 500 patients were treated, the hospital would have an unfavorable volume variance of $231,330. The calculation of this variance is shown below:

| | Volumes | | | Standard Product | |
|---|---|---|---|---|---|
| Product Name | Actual | Planned | Difference | Cost | Variance |
| DRG No. 139 | 500 − | 650 = | (150) | × $1,542.20 = | ($231,330) Unfavorable |

Mix variances represent the difference in the types of products being produced at a given volume level. Assume the hospital planned a total of 1,150 discharges: 650 discharges in DRG No. 139 at a cost of $1,542.20 and 500 discharges in DRG No. 140 at a cost of $1,950.10. If actual discharges were still 1,150, but consisted of 550 in DRG No. 139 and 600 in DRG No. 140, a shift of 100 discharges from a lower-cost product to a higher-cost product would have occurred. The impact of this mix vari-ance would be a cost variance of $40,790, calculated as follows:

| Product Name | Volumes | | | Standard Product Cost | Variance |
|---|---|---|---|---|---|
| | Actual | Planned | Difference | | |
| DRG No. 139 | 500 − | 650 = | (100) | × $1,542.20 = | ($154,220) Over |
| DRG No. 140 | 600 − | 500 = | 100 | × $1,950.10 = | $195,010 Under |
| Total | 1,150 | 1,150 | 0 | | $ 40,790 Under |

Mix variances are generally not regarded as either favorable or unfavorable. The actual mix of products is usually considered to be over or under forecast. Though costs may increase, reimbursements may increase in proportion, offsetting the increase in cost. However, under capitation payment systems, mix variances (for example, high-cost products exceeding forecasted levels) may significantly contribute to increasing costs and subsequently lower profits.

A treatment variance is the quantification of the difference between planned and actual resource consumption for a given product. For example, in DRG No. 139, three days of nursing care at Acuity Level 4 is the standard resource consumption. Assume a patient required only one Acuity Level 4 day. In this case, a favorable variance of two Acuity Level 4 days has occurred. Since each Acuity Level 4 day has a standard cost of $115.39, a favorable treatment variance of $230.78 has occurred for that procedure. All individual procedure variances within a product are calculated in this manner and then summed to arrive at a total product treatment variance. In Exhibit 3–8, an example of a treatment variance computation is presented.

Volume, mix, and treatment variances account for the changes between planned and actual hospital costs that are attributable to product-related concerns. Reports of such variances are generally used by top management and physicians.

## Performance Reporting on a Functional Level

Another function of a cost management system is to monitor and control the cost to produce a procedure. Unlike the case with products, the actual resources consumed in producing a day of nursing care or any other procedure are generally not individually captured. Rather, their costs are accumulated in general ledger subaccounts (for example, RN salaries, plastic supplies) across all procedures for a given period. Using the actual procedure count for a reporting period and extending it against each procedure's standard resource and cost profile, a total

**Exhibit 3–8** Example of a Product Treatment Variance Computation

Product Treatment Variance Report

Period: September 1 to September 30, 1985
Responsibility: J. Jones
# Cases: 23

Product No.:    DRG No. 139
Product Name:   Cardiac Arrhythmia & Conduction Disorders Age < 70 W/O C.C.

| Procedure Number/Name | Standard Procedure Usage | Actual Procedure Usage | Usage Variance | Standard Unit Cost | Cost Impact |
|---|---|---|---|---|---|
| Admission/discharge procedures | | | | | |
| 100101 Admission—normal | 1 | = 1 | 0 × | $ 26.19 | = $ 0 |
| 100109 Medical record processing | 1 | = 1 | 0 × | 42.12 | = 0 |
| 100110 Billing—Medicare | 1 | = 1 | 0 × | 19.85 | = 0 |
| Nursing procedures | | | | | |
| 300123 Nursing Care Level 1 | 1 | = 1 | (1) × | 43.13 | = (43.13) |
| 300223 Nursing Care Level 2 | 3 | = 3 | 0 × | 69.85 | = 0 |
| 300323 Nursing Care Level 3 | 4 | = 3 | 1 × | 88.42 | = 88.42 |
| 300423 Nursing Care Level 4 | 3 | = 1 | 2 × | 115.39 | = 230.78 |
| Day-of-stay procedures | | | | | |
| 20100 Normal meal | 17 | = 22 | (5) × | 8.79 | = (43.95) |
| 200410 Laundry/linen—medical | 9 | = 7 | 2 × | 3.38 | = 6.76 |
| 200950 Housekeeping—normal | 11 | = 9 | 2 × | 3.13 | = 6.26 |

Diagnostic and therapeutic procedures

| Code | Procedure | | | | | | | | | |
|------|-----------|---|---|---|---|---|---|---|---|---|
| 800422 | Chest x-ray pa/lat | 1 | — | 1 | = | 0 | × | 37.37 | = | 0 |
| 900123 | Lab CBC | 1 | — | 1 | = | 0 | × | 2.85 | = | 0 |
| 900124 | Lab electrolytes | 3 | — | 5 | = | (2) | × | 16.60 | = | (33.20) |
| 700011 | EKG—bedside | 1 | — | 1 | = | 0 | × | 38.99 | = | 0 |
| 600910 | IV therapy | 7 | — | 9 | = | (2) | × | 22.60 | = | (45.20) |
| | Total cost variance | | | | | | | | | $166.74 |

"earned" cost or flexed budget (standard costs extended by actual procedure volumes) for the cost center can be computed.

For example, if actual days of care provided were 1,400, 3,910, 4,404, and 6,300 for Acuity Levels 1 to 4, respectively, the nursing cost center in our example would earn $809,846 of variable costs. This is determined by multiplying each acuity level's standard variable cost per day by its actual volume. The earned costs would then be compared with the cost center's actual variable costs, as reported on the general ledger, to determine if the center incurred more or less expense than expected at the actual level of production. Exhibit 3–9 shows the calculation for this example.

It is important to note that this type of analysis is most appropriate for variable costs. Indirect (fixed) cost center costs, such as those for supervision and travel, are more discretionary expenditures that are generally unrelated to volumes. Cost center manager performance in controlling these costs is usually evaluated by comparing planned spending with actual spending levels. Similarly, overhead costs—costs that are typically beyond the control of cost center managers—should not be

**Exhibit 3–9** Example of a Cost Center Efficiency Variance Calculation

Cost Center Efficiency Variance

Cost Center: Medical Units
Period: Period ending September 30, 1985

| Procedure Number/Name | Actual Procedure Volumes | Standard Variable Unit Cost | Earned Variable Costs | Actual Variable Costs | Efficiency Variance |
|---|---|---|---|---|---|
| 300123 Nursing Care Level 1 | 1,400 × | $23.98 = | $ 33,572 | | |
| 300223 Nursing Care Level 2 | 3,910 × | 32.25 = | 126,098 | | |
| 300323 Nursing Care Level 3 | 4,404 × | 49.80 = | 219,319 | | |
| 300423 Nursing Care Level 4 | 6,300 × | 68.39 = | 430,857 | | |
| Totals | | | $809,846 | − $884,271 | = ($74,425) |

included in cost center performance reporting, even though they may be allocated to cost centers and then to procedures for full-absorption costing purposes.

Cost center performance reporting can occur at varying levels of detail. The example cited above looked at total cost center costs. Alternative types of reporting might include variances at natural expense classifications—salaries, benefits, and supplies; the general ledger subaccount level; or the job code level. A hospital can choose the detail level at which it reports, but increased detail has trade-offs that must be recognized; for example, small variances among job codes may net out to nil, increased data processing speed will produce degradation, and so on. In addition, general ledger subaccounts may have to be classified as either fixed or variable, and fixed and variable actual costs would have to be identified and recorded in the proper subaccount.

For certain types of expenses, further variance analysis may be provided. Beyond a total wage variance, an analysis of labor efficiency, focusing, for example, on earned versus actual hours or on the labor rate, calculated as planned versus actual hourly wage, may be provided. This preparation of this kind of supplemental variance analysis is contingent upon the capabilities of the hospital transaction (data collection) systems, such as the payroll system. While labor performance reporting may typically be provided, few hospitals have materials management systems to analyze supply costs beyond a total dollar variance. For example, material efficiency and purchase price variances will typically be long-term in development for most hospitals.

## SUMMARY

This overview outlines the generic concepts of cost management systems in hospitals. While great diversity may exist among hospital managers with regard to specific definitions, detail levels, and uses, a full-function cost management system will include all of the components described in this chapter. However, the generic concepts are modular, and hospitals may choose to implement only those modules that address their immediate needs.

The overall objectives and benefits of a full-function cost management system are summarized in Table 3–2. Hospitals may selectively choose to implement portions of a comprehensive system to provide them with the defined benefits that are most appropriate for their given circumstances.

Designing an effective cost management system at a given hospital involves two major challenges: (1) recognizing the unique needs and

**Table 3–2** Objectives and Benefits of a Cost Management System

| Product-Line Objectives | Product-Line Benefits |
| --- | --- |
| Maximization of net revenues | Using accurate cost data, more accurate bids on a per-product, discharge, or per-day basis can be prepared. |
| | Revenue and expense by line of business is provided. |
| | Third-party payer contracts can be evaluated for profitability performance. |
| Minimization of costs | Product resource consumption profiles can be reviewed and analyzed for reductions in length of stay or procedures. |
| | Physician performance can be compared with norms to evaluate clinical efficiency. |
| Maintenance of quality care | Excessive lengths of stay and costs can be analyzed as "outliers." |
| | Through a clinical database, the cost of complications can be identified. |
| Strategic planning to provide for future growth and rational decision making | Services can be expanded based on profitability through outreach programs, physician recruiting, marketing, and capital expenditures. |
| | Selective divesting can occur in costly and unprofitable product lines. |
| Development of depth in the management team | Hospital executives can improve management based on market needs. |
| | Product-line managers can promote their "business units" without day-to-day production concerns. |

| Functional (Cost Center) Objectives | Functional (Cost Center) Benefits |
| --- | --- |
| Increased productivity and minimization of costs | Initial standards development can reveal opportunities to streamline operations. |
| | Ongoing monitoring systems can evaluate performance and define accountability. |
| Improved planning and staffing | Cost center activity forecasts can be based on product volumes and standard resource consumption. |
| | Staffing levels can be initially based on demand forecast and flexed as demand changes. |

| Functional (Cost Center) Objectives | Functional (Cost Center) Benefits |
| --- | --- |
| Cost center facilities management supported by rational decision making | Demand for new services can be determined from product-line market analysis. |
| | The cost impact of new technologies can be quantified. |
| Better utilization and development of cost center managers' time | Managers need no longer be accountable for revenues or volumes—factors beyond their control. |
| | A sound basis of goal setting can be developed. |
| | Objective evaluation criteria can be established. |

capabilities of the hospital and (2) designing an appropriate "solution" to meet the defined needs with the identified capabilities. The intent of this and subsequent chapters is to guide the reader along a logical path in evaluating needs and designing and implementing appropriate cost management "solutions."

# chapter 4

# Practical Considerations of Implementation

## INTRODUCTION

The previous chapter presented the key concepts of a hospital cost management system and its functions and provided examples of those functions. However, it is unrealistic to assume that every hospital will want, need, or be able to purchase, develop, and support all of the defined functions. Therefore, it is extremely important that each hospital design, develop, and implement a cost management system that presents a "solution" based on the hospital's specific needs and situation.

Figure 4–1 depicts several factors that will influence the scope of a hospital-specific cost management system. To develop an appropriate cost management system, each of the factors shown must be examined

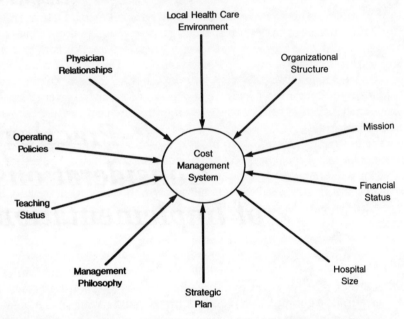

**Figure 4-1** Factors Influencing the Scope of a Hospital's Cost Management System

and its relative importance evaluated. For example, when looking at the hospital's local health care environment, the extent of competition typically will have a dramatic impact on the structure and timing of the cost management system. Hospitals in very competitive environments usually need an interim solution—for example, improved product pricing capabilities—to address their most urgent needs. Over time, these hospitals typically add other functions to provide a more sophisticated and detailed cost management system.

Similarly, financial status will play an important role in the type of system being implemented. Hospitals in financial distress will not require a complex system with an extended implementation timetable. Rather, they will require immediate operational improvements to ensure ongoing viability—such as productivity analyses.

Hospital size will also have an important effect on the sophistication level of the hospital's cost management system. On the one hand, smaller hospitals usually have a simpler organizational structure, with fewer tiers of management to oversee. Therefore, they may not feel the need for a highly sophisticated cost management system. On the other hand, larger hospitals and multifacility systems generally will need more sophisticated capabilities. Thus, for a hospital that is structured around strategic business units, the cost management system must provide the necessary cost information to help manage those units.

Mission and management philosophy are additional factors to consider within a hospital-specific cost management system. If, for example, the management philosophy is not aimed at clinical (physician/ treatment/product) monitoring, the hospital may want to orient its cost management system further toward budgeting and cost center performance monitoring.

If the hospital's mission is to provide a broad variety of services in a rural area, even if those services are not deemed profitable, the hospital may not need detailed product costing features for strategic planning purposes, but it may need cost center performance reporting in order to streamline operations. In other situations, certain operating policies, such as a no-lay-off policy, can have an impact on the effectiveness of a hospital's cost management system.

Teaching hospitals typically require a more sophisticated cost management system in order to identify accurately and to separate its direct and indirect teaching components—for research, teaching program evaluation, and competitive bidding purposes. In any case, the hospital's strategic plan will determine, to a major extent, the scope of the cost management system, since the system will be relied on to provide information for formulating and updating the plan.

Physician relationships also may have a dramatic impact on the selection and development of a cost management system. When implementing the system, support from all disciplines within the hospital is essential. When physicians are supportive, the development of standards is facilitated, product resource consumption profiles can be made more detailed and accurate, and the overall utility of the system will be enhanced. Finally, the complexity of the cost management system, its data processing capabilities, the personnel available to operate it, the hospital's education/training capabilities, and the time frame set by the hospital for implementation are all vital factors that will affect the nature and scope of each hospital's cost management system.

All of these factors have to be considered by the hospital when designing its unique cost management system. Each factor might be viewed either as a restriction on the scope of the system or as a factor that will help to determine the hospital's specific needs. If, for example, the time frame to design and implement the system is short, the system will likely not have a high degree of sophistication. In other cases, if hospital personnel are unfamiliar with the usage and interpretation of the reports produced by the system, the need for educational training will be critical to its usefulness as a source of information.

## COST MANAGEMENT SYSTEM NEEDS

It is difficult to indicate here, on a feature-by-feature basis, the specific cost management system needs of a particular hospital. However, we can at least suggest what the general needs of hospitals are likely to be, based on their size. In the following sections, we describe the typical needs for smaller hospitals (up to 200 beds), for medium-sized hospitals (200 to 500 beds), and for larger hospitals (over 500 beds) and multi-facility systems. These categories are not intended to represent absolute distinctions, but they do reflect general differences among hospitals with respect to cost management system needs. Within the categories, each hospital must examine its specific environment and structure in order to define its unique needs and to develop the appropriate cost management system to meet those needs.

### Smaller Hospital Needs

Hospitals with up to 200 beds typically do not need highly sophisticated cost management systems. Due to the size of their management teams and medical staff, a sophisticated capability to pinpoint areas of responsibility and span of control is generally not required, though this conclusion might not apply to smaller hospitals in highly competitive environments. Due to outside pressures, the latter hospitals may need more sophisticated cost management systems to provide the information needed to develop strategies in response to competition and to exercise greater control over their operations.

Smaller hospitals in less competitive environments are primarily concerned about maintaining volumes and controlling costs through gross measures, such as the use of an overall budget to control actual expenditures. Generally, their cost management systems must help them solve the following types of problems:

- improving cash flow/reserves
- developing bidding strategies
- strategic costing
- improving cost center productivity
- analyzing work flows

Controlling costs in smaller hospitals, to a greater extent than in larger hospitals, is often a basic strategic issue, since the portion of fixed costs in smaller hospitals is generally higher than larger hospitals due to unavailability of a large, skilled labor pool, a lower patient census, and so on. Thus, the number of minutes of technician time required to take a chest x-ray typically has little impact on a smaller hospital's costs. The overwhelming cost issues in smaller hospitals involve streamlining work flows, maintaining utilization levels, properly training staff, and using facilities appropriately.

However, a cost management system must provide all hospitals, regardless of size, with the appropriate information needed to manage their resources properly. If, for example, a cost center's productivity has to be improved, actual staffing levels must be compared with and monitored against expectations, based on budgeted, historical, or industry norms. In cost centers with poor performance compared with expectations, more detailed analyses of productivity, including cost center manager interviews and observations, should be performed. The goal here is not the development of procedure costs at a microlevel. Rather, it is the identification of macrolevel cost reductions or the possibilities for system improvement. Once a certain productivity level has been established, ongoing productivity monitoring can proceed through the cost management system to ensure compliance with expectations.

Smaller hospitals typically do not need full-function cost management software. However, they must still identify the cost management software, whether for a microcomputer or a minicomputer system, that best meets both short- and long-term needs of the hospital.

Other major objectives of smaller hospitals, not related to cost management, may involve becoming part of a multifacility system, creating joint ventures with physicians or other entities, or implementing other activities required to ensure the long-term survival of the hospital. In many cases, these moves may indeed become necessary, due to the major changes now occurring in the health care industry that are forcing smaller hospitals to reassess their role in the nation's health care delivery system. Since larger hospitals may seek to obtain their volumes from smaller hospitals through marketing, pricing, or outreach programs or by developing access arrangements with them, it is incumbent upon smaller hospitals, with generally fewer available resources, to assume a proactive position to ensure their ongoing success.

**Medium-Sized Hospital Needs**

Unlike smaller hospitals, medium-sized hospitals will generally need all of the components of a comprehensive cost management system, even though their implementation plans may be phased in over a number of years. Depending on their management orientation, medium-sized hospitals may initially implement a cost management system that reflects either of two basic orientations.

*Product-Line Orientation*

Medium-sized hospitals with a product-line management orientation are most concerned with strategic pricing and with evaluating product and physician performance, as a means of increasing revenues and controlling costs. This type of orientation is generally found in operating environments where competition is heated, where service areas are not expanding, or where management believes departmental costs are already as low as possible.

Cost management functions that best serve a product-line management orientation are the forecasting of product volumes and the reporting of product performance. Relative value units (RVUs) based on current production techniques and historical costs are generally used to determine product costs. Additionally, RVUs may be subsequently used to monitor the productivity of functional cost centers.

*Functional Orientation*

Medium-sized hospitals with a functional management orientation are most concerned with reducing and controlling production costs, rather than with evaluating product performance and marketing services. The operating environment of these hospitals is generally one of prolonged and declining inpatient utilization, poor financial performance, or a stagnant service area.

Cost management functions that are most appropriate in these circumstances are the determination of procedure costs and the reporting of cost center performance. The procedure-level standard costs that are determined are used as the basis for evaluating cost center manager performance. Additionally, these procedure cost standards may be used subsequently to determine the financial performance of the hospital's products.

Depending on their longer-term needs, medium-sized hospitals may gradually implement additional capabilities needed to upgrade to a full-function cost management system. Again, the urgency to do this will depend on the factors reflecting each individual hospital's environment.

**Larger Hospital and Multifacility System Needs**

Larger hospitals (more than 500 beds) need a full-function cost management system. Due to their size and complex organizational structures, these hospitals need to decentralize control and establish objective performance criteria. Therefore, their concerns involve performance reporting not only on a cost center level but also on a product level. To achieve better control and to facilitate strategic planning, larger hospitals require volume forecasting and budgeting capabilities as essential features of their cost management systems.

Since the scope of a cost management system and the related investment are typically greater for larger hospitals, it is very important for them to assess their needs correctly and then to select the appropriate computer software. Often, this will involve an initial implementation of short-term technology, such as a microcomputer application, until mainframe software can be closely evaluated or developed for long-term purposes.

Within the larger-hospital category, the needs of multifacility systems will vary, depending on their organizational structure, as reflected primarily in the level of centralization or decentralization. Within multifacility systems, the affiliations and organizational structures vary widely. A large number of multifacility systems have decentralized management with no line responsibility by a central body. For example, they may have religious affiliations, through a common congregation, but each entity may still operate autonomously. In other cases, the absence of consolidated financial statements and the existence of different computer systems at various locations indicate the extent of decentralization. In most instances, the individual hospitals within multifacility organizations have very diverse needs and constraints. Therefore, each must be evaluated separately to determine its probable need level.

In contrast to decentralized multifacility systems, centralized organizations, such as investor-owned systems, have many common needs and constraints—such as aggressive program pricing and similar computer hardware configurations. Often, one central person or committee is authorized to commit the entire organization. In this case, since the organization can be considered to be one large, though geographically dispersed, operating unit, its major concerns are often the same as those of larger hospitals. However, as a multifacility organization, it has at least one additional need—the need for comparative data. Each of its various facilities must have access to the procedural, cost center, and product standard data of the other facilities. To obtain maximum benefit from these data, multifacility systems usually require a comparative database. Cost management systems of multihospital organizations utilize such databases to provide additional benefits to specific end users and to the organization as a whole.

## DEFINING AND IMPLEMENTING A COST MANAGEMENT SYSTEM

The above discussion clearly indicates that a single generic cost management system will not meet the needs of all hospitals. To establish an effective cost management system, each hospital must thoroughly analyze all of the factors that determine its short- and long-term needs.

### A Generic Two-Step Approach

Yet, while there is no generic cost management solution for hospitals, there is a generic approach to the design of a cost management system. The approach consists of two major steps—system definition and implementation—each of which comprises a number of activities.

#### System Definition

System definition includes the activities identified in Figure 4–2. To guarantee the success of the cost management project, it is essential to organize a task force to lead the enterprise and serve as the key decision-making body. Next, education programs should be conducted for hospital personnel, the board of trustees, and the physicians. As end users of the cost management system, each of these groups must acquire an understanding of the advantages and benefits that a cost management system can provide. This will help to strengthen the commitment and cooperation of these groups during the implementation phase. Following these basic activities, the hospital has to assess its specific needs in the light of its existing information and transaction systems. Based on the result of this needs and systems assessment, the conceptual design can be developed and the necessary computer hardware/software can be selected.

#### Implementation

The second step toward the realization of the cost management system is implementation, which includes the activities identified in Figure 4–3. The first task in the implementation process is to install the requisite computer hardware and to customize the appropriate software. This may require modifications in the existing transaction systems, including the customizing of its reports. To guarantee effective operation and use of the system by end users, the implementation process must be combined with extensive user training. Once this has been

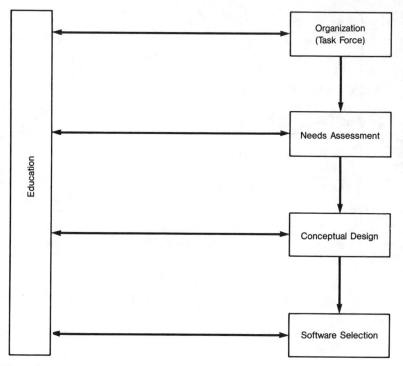

**Figure 4–2** System Definition

done, the processes of data gathering, entry, and verification can be initiated to finish the implementation phase.

### Benefits of a Two-Step Approach

Based on their specific needs, it might not be necessary for all hospitals to go through every phase of this generic approach. If a hospital decides, based on its needs assessment and the conceptual design of its cost management system, that its current computer system and software meet its needs, it will obviously not have to select and implement new computer equipment and software. In other cases, it may be unnecessary to customize new software to current transaction systems because the software is from the same vendor and therefore interfaces may be prepackaged.

In any case, the two-step approach provides several benefits. First, it ensures a practical, hospital-specific solution that is responsive to the hospital's unique situation and consistent with its mission and goals.

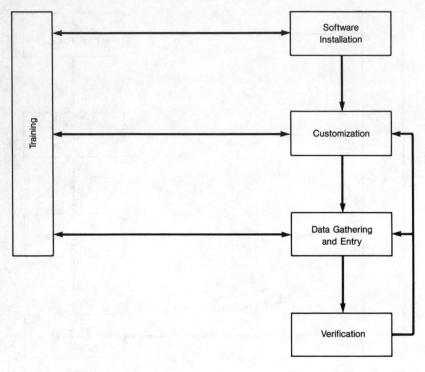

**Figure 4–3** Implementation

Second, it involves hospital employees, directors, and clinicians and thus promotes a committed, comprehensive, and coordinated effort. Third, by going through a needs-determination process, the involved personnel can gain important insights that will expedite implementation. For example, the process might show that the hospital's real need is immediate cost savings and that, therefore, strategic resizing rather than cost management is the most pressing activity to undertake. Also, in the process, it might become obvious that the hospital has to improve its strategic planning efforts or that a long-term performance-based incentive system should be implemented. Another consequence might be a decision by the hospital—based on the review of its operations—to streamline operations in selected departments before implementing the cost management system. Each of these activities can take place before, during, or after the implementation of the cost management system, depending on the hospital's specific needs, their urgency, and the available resources.

## SUMMARY

In designing and implementing its cost management system, each hospital must chart its own course. The ultimate success of any undertaking often rests with the proper identification and understanding of the various factors and limitations involved. In implementing a cost management system, it is thus imperative that caution be exercised and that the proper steps be executed to ensure a successful outcome.

# part II

# DEVELOPING A COST MANAGEMENT SYSTEM

# chapter 5

# Defining the System

## INTRODUCTION

As noted in the previous chapter, system definition is a critical component in the formulation of a cost management system that will be responsive to a hospital's specific needs. In this chapter, we detail the tasks required to determine a hospital's specific needs and their priority (urgency). Once these are determined, a series of activities can be implemented to define and document the cost management system structure (inputs, required calculations, and outputs) required to meet the hospital's short- and long-term requirements. Based on the outcome of these activities, the requisite cost management software can be properly evaluated and selected.

## SYSTEM DEFINITION ACTIVITIES

The logical sequence of activities during system definition is shown in the following five steps:

1. organization
2. education
3. needs assessment
4. conceptual design
5. software selection

### Organization

The first step in defining the cost management system is to organize a task force of hospital personnel (and an outside consultant, if appropriate) to serve as the key decision-making body and catalyst of the cost management project. It is recommended that the task force consist of no more than eight to ten people. By thus limiting the size of the task force, key decisions can generally be reached more quickly, increasing the probability that the cost management project will meet its predefined timetable. The following should be considered as potential members of the task force:

- chief operating officer
- chief financial officer
- chief information officer
- director of nursing
- controller
- cost accountant
- management engineer
- ancillary cost center managers (typically one or two)
- physicians (for example, chief of medical staff)

It is important to have a senior executive, such as the chief operating officer, serve on the task force. This reinforces the commitment the hospital has to the cost management project and demonstrates that it is a hospitalwide—not merely a finance department—effort. Additionally, the director of nursing should be encouraged to serve on the task force, since nursing services typically represent 30 to 40 percent of a hospital's labor costs.

The second organizational step is to appoint a task force project director. This person will assume day-to-day responsibility for the project. The qualifications of the task force project director should include:

- familiarity with the hospital's organizational structure and clinical services
- familiarity with the hospital's financial reporting and accompanying support systems (for example, payroll, case mix)
- familiarity with external markets for the hospital's services, such as the Medicare Prospective Payment System, preferred provider organizations, major employers, and health maintenance organizations

It also is recommended that the task force project director position be established as a full-time responsibility to ensure that tasks are completed within predefined deadlines.

**Education**

To begin the actual definition of the cost management system, several task force orientation sessions should be conducted. The objectives of these sessions should be to:

- provide a common understanding of cost management concepts and applications
- reinforce the responsibilities of task force members
- define the process of establishing a cost management system as a means to meet specific short- and long-term needs of the hospital

The orientation meetings will normally be led by the project director. Initially, broad cost management system concepts, such as the key system outputs and the inputs required to produce those outputs, are discussed. Detailed requirements are not discussed by the task force as a whole.

Orientation sessions also should be conducted for the hospital's management team, board of directors, medical staff, and cost center managers, as appropriate. These sessions generally take place after the structure of the hospital's cost management system is defined. Again, an overview of the concepts, outputs, and benefits of the cost management system should be presented. The presentations should be tailored to show how the cost management system supports the needs, responsibilities, and functions of each group.

## Needs Assessment

For most hospitals, a full-function cost management system is necessary to meet their long-range objectives and information requirements. However, due to immediate needs (for example, the need to respond to an HMO contract bid) or other circumstances, many hospitals choose to implement initially only one or two cost management system applications. Commonly encountered circumstances that may lead to a phased implementation of applications include the following:

- The hospital may not have the computer hardware capabilities or capacity to process all of the desired cost management systems applications.
- The hospital's existing transactions systems (for example, payroll) may not capture the data elements required to support fully the projected cost management system.
- The hospital may be currently undertaking major renovations or replacements in certain areas.
- Implementation of all of the functions simultaneously may overwhelm end users.
- Adequate staff may not be available to carry out the requisite data-gathering and implementation tasks.

### Four Generic Categories

To determine the hospital's specific needs and the corresponding priorities for cost management applications to meet those needs, key end users of the cost management system should be identified and interviewed. These individuals are generally represented by:

- top management
- physicians
- cost center managers
- product-line managers

Generally, 15 to 20 individuals provide an adequate basis to document and assign priorities to a hospital's needs. The most efficient and consistent way to document the hospital's needs is to develop a needs assessment questionnaire. This questionnaire should include needs and objectives in the four generic categories presented in Figure 5–1. These involve:

1. responding to competitive market pressures
2. planning and controlling functional cost center resources
3. monitoring physician resource management
4. planning and managing by product line

In the following sections, we present a brief description of each category, its corresponding internal or external environmental factors, and its data requirements.

**Competitive Market Pressures.** Response to competitive market pressures becomes a need when hospitals are required to formulate and submit pricing schedules to retain a portion of their business (for example, a Blue Cross or HMO contract) or to compete for total patient markets that have been fragmented (for example, an employer PPO contract).

The more successful responses to competitive pressures are based on accurate total and marginal cost information at both the procedure and

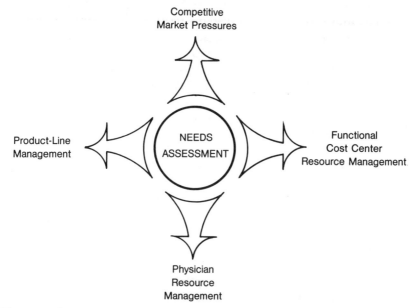

**Figure 5–1** Categories of Needs Assessment

product levels. With this type of information, a sound basis can be formed for developing competitive prices and estimating the contract's profitability. Also, many contracts require that pricing schedules reflect some type of case mix measure (for example, obstetric services). This necessitates a case mix system that can accept and process patient classification attribute criteria.

The following are appropriate questionnaire items in this category:

- Are you losing market share? If yes, can you determine how much, why, and in which services and clinical areas?
- Do you monitor the activity and profitability of your current medical service contracts? If yes, how (level of detail, accuracy, etc.)?
- Are HMOs prevalent in your service area? If yes, what is the status of your current HMO opportunities?
- Are you perceived as a low- or high-cost provider?

**Functional Cost Center Resource Management.** The planning and controlling of functional cost center resources generally becomes a need when various operational circumstances have affected the hospital's financial stability. These circumstances may include large losses over multiple periods, continued declining utilization, or the submission and acceptance of a medical service contract at a low profit margin. Hospitals may also need new systems to plan and control resources if existing systems are regarded as inadequate and ineffective.

The planning component involves projecting activities, resources, and costs at various levels of utilization and inflation to set the hospital's overall profitability and goals. The control component involves the calculation and reporting of variances to monitor an individual's performance in achieving that individual's objectives and in controlling costs during the fiscal year.

Successful implementation of a cost management system to meet this need helps a hospital reduce its operating costs, become more competitive in price, and increase its profitability.

The following are appropriate questionnaire items in this category:

- Are your current planning (budgeting) systems and methodologies adequate? If not, what would you change, and why?
- Do you currently have a productivity system in place? If yes, is it well-accepted by department managers?
- Do you currently have a patient classification system in place? If yes, is it well-accepted by nursing managers?

The monitoring of physician resource management has been a procedure of last resort for most hospitals. Usually, these hospitals are unwilling to work with physicians for fear of losing admissions and control of the clinical aspect of the business. However, today more hospitals are discovering that comparative resource utilization information, especially on a physician-to-physician basis, helps physicians initiate more consistent and effective treatment protocols and thereby reduce costs.

**Physician Resource Management.** The monitoring of physician resource usage requires a case mix system with a comparative reporting capability and access to regional or national treatment protocol databases. In addition, cost information must be related to each procedure that makes up a treatment variance. In this way, the dollar impact (favorable or unfavorable) of current or new treatment practices can be quantified. Ideally, to perform this function, a case mix system that accepts procedural cost information and integrates this information with user-defined case types is preferable.

The following are appropriate questionnaire items in this category:

- Do your physicians desire better information regarding their treatment practices? If yes, in what form?
- Does your current case mix system have the capability to provide physicians with the information they want?
- Has the hospital or its physicians organized a pcer review committee? If yes, what are the major functions of this committee, and what has been its effect on physicians?

**Product-Line Management.** Planning and managing by product line become a need when a hospital's existing organizational structure is inadequate for planning, marketing, reporting, and clinical management purposes. Product-line management information needs are generally met by a cost management system that incorporates accurate procedural cost information and a product-forecasting and performance-monitoring application. If the hospital is organized in this way to respond more effectively to its markets, increased utilization and profitability should result.

The following are appropriate questionnaire items in this category:

- How many different product lines do you anticipate forming? Will these be implemented simultaneously, or will they be staggered?

- Does your current case mix system have the capability to meet your product-line needs?
- Have you discussed product-line management with your physicians and cost center managers? If yes, what was their reaction?

*The Assessment Process*

Every hospital will agree that each of these needs and objectives is, at least nominally, important to its institution. However, the success of the needs assessment process depends on a determination of the degree of importance (priority) placed on each objective.

The needs assessment interviews should be conducted by the task force project director and/or outside consultants. In this way, insights regarding cost management concepts and the hospital's current operating/reporting structure can be documented, while at the same time clarifying the hospital's cost management objectives.

After all the needs assessment interviews and questionnaires are completed, the responses are summarized and presented to the task force. The task force uses this information to confirm the objectives and priorities of the cost management system applications. The interviews and the confirmation of objectives and priorities by the task force should normally be completed within three weeks.

**Conceptual Design**

After identifying the scope and depth of the hospital's needs, the conceptual design of the cost management system must be documented. The purpose of the conceptual design is to build on the needs assessment to:

- evaluate practical options
- identify constraints
- establish timetables to develop the desired cost management capabilities

*Components*

The components of the conceptual design are:

- desired outputs and report distribution
- required underlying calculations
- input data elements

- interfaces with existing systems
- system constraints

**Desired Outputs and Report Distribution.** The desired outputs and report distribution are tools used by the hospital management to make key business decisions. The relevant process should include a listing of the required reports, identification of their distribution frequency and their content and uses, and the development of prototype report formats. The reports should be understood by and acceptable to the managers who receive them. This generally entails reviewing the prototype report formats with a sampling of report end users (for example, cost center managers) and then revising them as necessary, based on the comments given.

**Underlying Calculations.** The underlying calculations required to produce each report should be documented. This serves two purposes. At a minimum, the documentation will assist in defining the required input data elements of the cost management system. Additionally, since many cost management software systems provide no (or only limited) standard reporting, input data element identification can assist the hospital by serving as a basis for determining functional specifications in the programming of hospital-specific, custom reports.

**Input Data Elements.** The input data elements consist of two distinct sets: standard and actual. Examples of standard input data elements are:

- standard procedure resource and cost profiles
- standard product resource consumption profiles
- standard charges and payments for each procedure and product

Examples of actual input data elements are:

- actual procedure and product volumes
- actual cost center resources and costs incurred
- actual product resource consumption

**Interfaces with Existing Systems.** The next step is to determine the sources of the input data elements required by the cost management system. Standard input data elements are generally derived from a combination of special studies (for example, time and motion) and existing transaction systems data (for example, payroll data for current labor rates and materials management data for current supply unit costs).

Actual input data elements, required for standards maintenance and performance reporting, are derived solely from existing (or planned) hospital transaction systems (for example, from billing for actual procedure volumes and from general ledger for actual costs incurred by a cost center). Normally, the hospital's existing transaction systems include:

- general ledger
- payroll
- materials management
- patient classification
- medical records
- patient billing
- fixed asset ledger
- statistical data gathering

Each of these transaction systems should be documented to determine the existence of required input data elements and the means to interface them with the cost management system.

In documenting each transaction system, four issues are critical:

1. General data availability—Are the data captured?
2. Data quality—Do the data contain significant errors?
3. Direct transfer potential—Is the transfer computerized?
4. Data manipulation requirements—At what level of detail do the data exist? Are the reporting periods consistent with other transaction system reporting periods?

**System Constraints.** If any of the transaction systems cited above do not currently exist at the hospital, or if the data they currently capture are of questionable integrity or represent inappropriate content, certain outputs of the cost management system may not be fully realized. This situation will require that the deficiencies in data collection be corrected or that the relevant transaction system or systems be subsequently implemented. For example, if the hospital wishes to incorporate patient acuity information into the cost management system and does not currently have a patient classification system in place, the inclusion of this input data element into the cost management system will have to be deferred until the requisite patient classification system is established.

Ideally, input data elements from the hospital's transaction systems are transferred electronically through reformat/interface programs to the cost management system. The input data elements may have to be formatted, to ensure that actual and standard data are consistent and comparable, before performance reporting or standards maintenance applications can be executed. In addition to formatting and transferring input data elements, where the specific input data elements do not exist but where the underlying data elements needed to calculate it do exist, the reformat/interface programs may also be required to recalculate (manipulate) the data elements (for example, average wage rates).

The development of specific reformat/interface programs is based on the implementation priority of each cost management system application, the cost benefit of developing and maintaining the program, and the availability of required data elements currently captured by existing hospital transaction systems. In the case of a transaction system software constraint, a short-term solution—such as no interface with the materials management system—will be utilized; in the long term, an upgrading of the materials management system may be considered. In other instances, hospitals may have a data-processing hardware constraint, affecting hardware capacity or hardware configurations (some systems may involve timesharing, others may be based completely in-house). In such cases, the constraint should be evaluated carefully to determine the realistic options available to the hospital in the short- and mid-term.

## Documentation

To facilitate the transaction system documentation process, documentation questionnaires should be used to gather the relevant data. After the questionnaires are completed, the responses should be summarized and reviewed. Issues that may indicate obstacles in the realization of the cost management system or one of its components (for example, the unavailability of payroll data by skill level or an inability to interface due to systems incompatibility) should be presented to the task force. Short- and long-term solutions to resolve each issue can then be agreed upon and documented.

After all the relevant tasks are completed (organization, education, needs assessment, and transaction systems review), an outline report documenting the conceptual structure of the cost management system should be prepared. Optionally, a formal conceptual design document can be prepared, but this should be done only if the cost management system is to be custom programmed or if the hospital wishes to use the conceptual design as an educational document for hospital managers.

The conceptual design document serves two purposes. First, it organizes and presents the details of the hospital's cost management system. These details generally include the following three elements:

1. the hospital's short- and long-term cost management objectives
2. the system's structure:

   • input data elements
   • processing calculations
   • outputs (reports or data files)

3. data collection requirements and issues:

   • existence
   • detail
   • interface capabilities

Second, the conceptual design document provides the basis for selecting or developing computer software and for formulating a work plan to capture the required input data elements.

**Software Selection**

The conceptual design provides the hospital with a documented system definition. At this point, the hospital must either select the software that best meets its needs, subject to identified constraints, or must internally develop the software required to meet its needs. In either case, the software component of the cost management solution may serve either interim or long-term needs, depending on the hospital's specific environment and objectives. In some instances, the hospital may opt for a comprehensive, integrated, mainframe-based cost management system.

In any event, before deciding on software, the hospital should identify and evaluate the cost management software options currently available in the marketplace. This is very important, since the software available to support some or all of the objectives of cost management in hospitals changes very rapidly. For example, several years ago, most so-called cost management software was limited to a handful of timesharing budgeting systems. Then a plethora of case mix systems—with widely varying capabilities—came on the market, in conjunction with a number of cost-determination products. To select the appropriate software to meet its cost management needs, hospital management should follow the steps outlined in Figure 5–2.

Rather than mass-mailing requests for proposals, hospitals should first review preliminary cost management system information, such as that found in marketing literature. In this part of the selection process, the following considerations are pertinent:

- The software's capability to provide identified outputs
- The software's fit within existing constraints
- Preliminary cost estimates for the software system
- The technology used by the software

Once the population of software systems has been narrowed down to those that clearly meet the hospital's general criteria, efforts should be focused on such tactical concerns as:

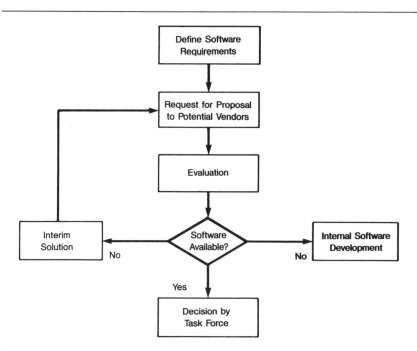

**Figure 5–2** Software Selection

- resources required for operation
- vendor reputation and support
- total system cost

This step is important in defining the software requirements and in clarifying the specific objectives it should achieve.

The hospital should then prepare a formal Request For Proposal (RFP) that addresses all of the relevant strategic and tactical issues through a comprehensive set of inquiries. In the RFP, each requirement of the cost management system should be documented clearly and comprehensively.

The next step is to summarize and interpret the responses to the RFP, as a basis for evaluating the commonalities and differences of each software system and its match to the cost management system's conceptual design. To facilitate both the preparation of an RFP and the comparative analysis of software alternatives indicated by the responses, a standard comprehensive software evaluation form should be used. The evaluation format should include adequate explanations instead of simple yes/no answers. At this point, the selection process should have narrowed the choices down to no more than three potential vendors. Presentations and reference site visits should then be arranged as necessary.

After the vendor presentations and site visits are completed, the key points and impressions of each software product regarding its ability to meet the requirements of the cost management system should be outlined. A task force meeting can then be held to review the key aspects of each system and select the appropriate vendor package.

Occasionally, the cost management software required to meet a hospital's needs will be unavailable. This may be due to inappropriate hardware configurations, the inadequacy of microcomputer applications, or mismatches between available packages and the hospital's system requirements, resources, and budget. In such cases, the hospital may have to develop its cost management system internally.

Several potential problems may arise when a hospital chooses to develop a system internally:

- If the system is not viewed as a joint venture between end users and the development team, the result may be poor communication and a system that does not match the user's requirements.
- Internal development of software takes longer, and the cost is usually greater than that for software purchased externally.

- The systems may be created without benefit of an appropriate development methodology. This can lead to poor and inconsistent project management, quality, and documentation.

Compounding these problems, the hospital may have limited human, hardware, and software resources. Yet, once a hospital commits itself to the development of a system internally, it assumes responsibility for maintenance, support, and the avoidance of backlogs. Thus, though internal development might provide an interim solution in some cases, most hospitals should carefully consider the advantages of customizing purchased software and thereby avoid the extended manpower costs and delays of internal development.

## SUMMARY

Hospitals are faced with a significant challenge when they design, develop, and implement a cost management system. Because the cost management system will inevitably become the cornerstone of the hospital's decision-support systems, the process of its selection must be based on a logical sequence of events. Some hospitals respond to the challenge by soliciting proposals without adequately defining their system needs and constraints. Adherence to the carefully devised plan will minimize the risk of purchasing and installing a cost management system that does not address the hospital's needs or requires excessive resources to operate.

# chapter 6

# *Implementing the System*

## INTRODUCTION

Once the system has been defined, the hospital will have a thorough documentation of its cost management needs, a conceptual design of a cost management system to meet those needs, a selection of (or a development plan for) software, and a general timetable for implementation to respond to the conceptual design. This chapter addresses the next phase of activities, those relating to the implementation of the cost management system.

## THE IMPLEMENTATION PLAN

Depending on the vendor and software selected, whether a microcomputer or a mainframe product, the implementation process for a cost management system may vary greatly. In some cases, as noted earlier, the hospital may decide to develop its own software application to meet its specific needs, either because no software products are compatible with its hardware or because the functions of the available products do not meet its needs. In any event, while the process may vary for purchased software and in-house development, a generic five-step implementation process is advisable. (For purposes of the following discussion, we assume that products developed in-house are at the same stage of completion as purchased products.)

Five specific activities are necessary to implement a cost management system:

1. software installation
2. customization
3. training
4. data gathering and data entry
5. verification

The cost management task force should develop an implementation plan to address each of these five activities. Based on the conceptual design and software selection process, the hospital should understand the resources—manpower, data, and hardware—required to implement the selected system. The implementation plan should then address how existing hospital resources will be allocated, or how additional resources (for example, consultants) will be obtained, to implement the system within the desired time frame.

In developing the plan, the task force must address specifically the issues of day-to-day resource availability in the finance, management engineering, and data processing departments. This will require an evaluation of the total resources available—resources that may be in contention with other projects—and the relative availability of each to the cost management project. Usually, the requisite resources will not be available and allocable to the project, and consultants will be required to assist in implementation efforts. Indeed, as the initial implementation efforts begin to exceed the ongoing maintenance requirements, the use of consultants may be completely cost-justified.

The precise level of involvement of external consultants in each of the implementation activities will depend on several key variables:

- the availability of qualified hospital personnel
- the level of support provided by the vendor

- the sophistication of the application
- the desired timetable

**Software Installation**

Generally, software installation can involve either a mainframe or minicomputer installation or a microcomputer installation. Most vendors of mainframe cost management systems provide software installation services as well. Generally, the vendor will tailor its system's job control language (or equivalent) to operate in the particular hospital's environment. This process may be performed either on-site or in the vendor's facility. The vendor will either physically install and test its system at the hospital site or will provide instructions and simulations for installation at some central site.

Similarly, microcomputer software vendors may provide either documentation or assistance, or both, in the installation of their products. If they do not provide assistance, and the hospital is not familiar with microcomputers, external consultants may perform the installation process. This typically involves loading the system software from vendor computer disks onto the hospital's computer. If assistance is needed in this process, it should be provided by consultants with experience in microcomputers and, preferably, with the specific vendor's package.

Regardless of the type of software purchased, hospitals have the right to expect complete software installation support from the vendor. When this is not available, the hospital will have to consider additional costs involved in engaging external data systems consultants or in the use of internal staff time to implement the installation.

**Customization**

For hospitals purchasing a mainframe-based cost management system, some degree of customization will be required. While the policies of individual software vendors vary as to which organization should assume responsibility for programming the customizations, the responsibility to define the required customization rests with the hospital.

Customization may be required to:

- interface the cost management system with the hospital's transaction processing systems
- produce output reports
- modify the standard system operation

The first two of these types of customization are the most common and are often required to make the system functional at a given hospital. In the first type, the interfaces do not alter the operational source code of the software product, but rather serve to enhance the individual data-entry and reporting functions of the standard product for the particular hospital. The third type of customization involves a direct change in the system's operational source code, thereby changing its computational or data-formatting characteristics. Such changes often void the warranties on the software. Indeed, to maintain the integrity of their systems and to provide uniform support, most vendors strongly discourage alterations in their system source codes. The three types of customizations are described in greater detail in the following sections.

*Interfaces*

In the system definition phase, the conceptual design identifies the appropriate interfaces required between the cost management system and the hospital's transaction processing systems. In the implementation phase, these interfaces must be programmed. This requires the preparation of detailed specifications or data element analyses. The specifications for each desired interface must detail each data element to be transferred between the systems, indicate the location and format of the data in each system, and document any specific data manipulation (for example, calculations or format changes) that is required. While the preparation of such detailed interface specifications is time-consuming, it reduces both programming time and the risk of error in the programs themselves.

The exact format of the interface specifications will be unique to each combination of transaction and cost management systems being interfaced. A hypothetical example of an interface specification between a payroll system and a cost management system is presented in Exhibit 6–1.

Once the specifications are completed, the interfaces may be programmed and tested. The responsibility for writing and testing the programs will vary, depending on the software vendor. A few vendors offer the interface programming as part of the installation process; some offer the programming as an additional-fee service. Still others do not write any interfaces; instead, they provide high-level languages and data dictionaries to assist hospitals in writing the interface programs themselves.

*Output Reports*

Cost management systems differ greatly in the way they provide information to the users. Some systems offer an extensive array of pre-

**Exhibit 6–1**  An Example of Interface Specifications

Interface Specifications

Payroll system file name: REGISTER.DATA
Cost management system file name: ACTUALPR.DATA

| | Cost Management System Data Elements | | Payroll System Data Elements | | | Conversion Rules | |
|---|---|---|---|---|---|---|---|
| *Description* | *Length* | *Type* | *Starting Position* | *Length* | *Type* | *Payroll* | *Cost Management* |
| Department | 10 | AN | 2 | 6 | N | | Right justify, zero fill |
| Labor class | 6 | AN | 8 | 3 | N | | Right justify, zero fill |
| Worked hours | | N | 15 | 10(8.2) | N | Sum each occurrence within cost center and labor class | |
| Actual pay rate | 5(3.2) | N | — | — | — | Compute on costs divided by hours | |
| Total costs | 11(9.2) | N | 72* | 11(9.2) | N | *Obtain from General Ledger file for each combination of cost center and labor class | |

| LABOR CLASS | ACCOUNT SUFFIX |
|---|---|
| 10 | 100 |
| 20 | 110 |
| 30 | 120 |
| 40 | 130 |
| 50 | 140 |

programmed standard reports; others offer a limited number of reports with some ad hoc reporting capabilities. Still others offer few or no standard reports, choosing instead to provide high-level, custom report-writing software. From a strategic standpoint, hospitals must evaluate whether a given system can provide the reports documented in the conceptual design. If custom reporting is required, the conceptual design can serve as the basis for the programming specifications. Here again, the cost of programming custom reports—either in programming fees or staff time—must be considered in evaluating the system's cost.

*System Modifications*

Occasionally, a software system will need system modifications to perform in accordance with the conceptual design. Generally, changes in a purchased system's internal operations should not be made because it will limit the vendor's ability to provide support and furnish updates. When changes are required, they should be identified in the software selection process, and their cost and impact on future support should be evaluated. In general, when making such changes, it is recommended that hospitals do not change the system source code.

**Training**

Most software vendors include technical training as part of the installation process, at a cost that either is already included in the software price or is stipulated as an additional fee. However, such training is generally related to system operation by data-processing personnel, not to actual end-user applications. Some vendors do provide limited, generic, end-user training, usually at a central training facility, again, either as a service for a separate fee or as a "throw-in" with the software purchase.

The hospital must carefully evaluate the training level being offered by the software vendor. Nonconsulting vendors generally do not get involved with hospital-specific training issues; instead they offer generic operational training courses. Yet, the ultimate success of implementing a cost management system is dependent on its effective use by hospital managers. Therefore, end-user training has to be provided. This training should address a number of key concerns—including what reports are available (how often), how to read and interpret the reports, how to develop the relevant policies and procedures for end-user understanding, and how to establish the policies and procedures for using the system's outputs.

End-user training should separately address specific groups, such as top management, product-line managers, physicians, and functional cost center managers. A presentation should also be made to the board of trustees regarding the system's structure and reporting capabilities and the board's responsibilities regarding the application of the cost management data, as they affect the board's function, as well as the functions of other levels and types of hospital personnel.

The training aspect of implementation is vital to the success of the cost management system. Since most hospitals do not possess all the necessary expertise and facilities needed to provide comprehensive and extensive training, they are usually forced to look to outside sources to meet the need.

**Data Collection and Data Entry**

Data collection and data entry activities are necessary in all hospital cost management systems, regardless of the software selected. Some data collection is accomplished through the conceptual design and interface-programming steps. However, the majority of inputs usually have to be developed from the ground up. This process entails the establishment of standard procedure cost profiles and product resource consumption profiles and the gathering of various statistics.

The establishment of standard cost profiles at both procedure and product levels is a complex task, yet it is integral to the successful implementation of the cost management system. While classified as an implementation task because of its complexity and time requirements, data gathering should actually begin as the conceptual design phase is drawing to a close.

To initialize the system, procedure and product profiles will be based on, or verified against, some control period data (historical or budgeted). Once the cost management system has been run, the results should again be verified against the control period. Each cost center's performance should be analyzed to confirm that earned costs are properly computed, on a test basis, and that the calculated variances are reasonable, given the cost center's current operating characteristics. A similar process should be followed in analyzing product performance.

Besides verifying system accuracy against a control period, the cost management task force must become familiar with the operations of the system and its results, as a basis for presentation to other hospital personnel. Upon distribution of the initial performance reports, the task force is likely to be called upon to explain certain unusual results. At this point, to maintain user confidence in the task force and the system, the task force must be fully informed as to the specific derivation and meaning of those results. Because of the complexity of the software implementation process, it is critical that user confidence be maintained. In hospitals that are developing a comprehensive cost management system, the standard-setting process may take 6 to 12 months or longer, depending on the resources available and the standard-setting methodology chosen. (The following chapters address these topics in depth.)

Because the establishment of standard procedure cost profiles and product resource consumption profiles is a very complex task, requiring specialized expertise and time-consuming and organizationally sensitive work, hospitals may not be able to or may not want to utilize their own staff for this purpose. By comparison, other data-gathering and data-entry procedures are more routine in nature, involving simply the gathering of the various data elements required to operate the cost management system.

### Verification

Upon implementation, cost management systems are highly susceptible to the reporting of erroneous results. The vast amounts of quantitative data—statistics, account balances, and so on—that are transferred and processed expose the system to a high risk of clerical and transactional error. Additionally, the existence of qualitative or subjective data—such as standards—in the system creates the risk of invalid conclusions or faulty data arising from properly computed results. This, in turn, can result in poor or inappropriate decision making. Thus, it is important in this final phase of the implementation process to track system results, to reconcile results with expectations, and to audit on a sample basis the validity of the system's reporting statistics.

### SUMMARY

The implementation process will vary with each hospital, depending on the computer hardware involved and the software product selected. In any case, regardless of the sophistication or technology of the selected system, implementation will be a significant and sensitive activity. Accordingly, a logical step-by-step approach should be tailored to the selected software. The goal is to implement an accurate, meaningful, and credible cost management system in a reasonable period of time, and with knowledgeable and interested system end users.

# chapter 7

# Setting Procedure Standard Cost Profiles

## INTRODUCTION

As indicated in the previous chapter, a major activity in the implementation phase of a cost management system involves the development of the appropriate data to enter into the system. There are two major data collection activities to be performed: (1) the development of procedure standard cost profiles and (2) the development of product resource consumption profiles. In this chapter, we address the first of these activities. The second activity is discussed in the following chapter.

Individual procedure resource profiles and cost standards are the building blocks of the product costing, performance-monitoring, and budgeting applications of a cost management system. The reports produced by these applications are reviewed and relied on by hospital executives to commit scarce resources, evaluate clinical services, evaluate individual performances, and augment strategic marketing decisions. Thus, a thorough understanding of the key issues and methodologies in gathering procedural resource and cost standard information is vital to the accuracy and reliability of the cost management system. The development of such information requires a thorough commitment by the hospital. The setting of procedure resource and cost standards is the most intensive and time-consuming part of the implementation process for a cost management system. If the hospital does not want to involve itself in this process or does not have the resources to do the required work, external assistance should be sought.

At the procedural level, several types of data must be gathered to implement the cost management system:

- individual procedure standard resource and cost data
- indirect cost center standard resource and cost data
- statistical allocation data

This chapter addresses the steps that are necessary to develop this information. It walks the reader through each step, as reflected in the components depicted in Figure 7–1.

## ORGANIZATION OF DATA-COLLECTION EFFORTS

In the data-gathering process, several organizational tasks need to be performed:

- assignment of cost centers
- selection of a control period
- classification of general ledger subaccounts into fixed-versus-variable categories
- calculation of control totals

### Assignment of Cost Centers

First, each hospital cost center should be assigned to one of these functional categories:

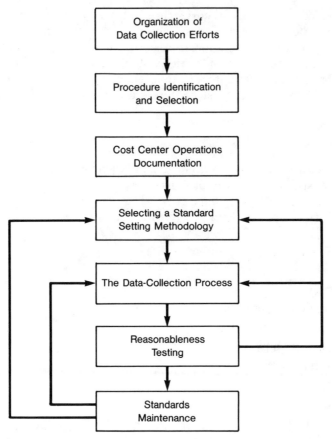

**Figure 7–1** The Data Collection Process

- direct patient care
- patient care support
- general overhead
- medical education

Hospital personnel involved in the cost center categorization process generally include the task force project director and the hospital's reimbursement specialist. Over the short term, apart from the above categorization, it may be necessary to classify cost centers as either revenue-producing or allocated. In this way, costing and data-gathering requirements may be simplified to meet immediate implementation goals.

The above four-part categorization helps to identify the costing approach to be used for each cost center and to determine which cost centers will need to have allocation statistics developed. A list of the hospital's cost centers usually can be obtained through the hospital's financial reporting system (for example, general ledger). Definitions and examples of the various cost centers are presented in the following sections.

*Direct Patient Care*

Direct patient care cost centers generally perform "hands on" nursing, diagnostic, therapeutic, or consultation procedures. Historically, most of these cost centers have charged for the services they perform. Direct patient care cost centers typically include:

- medical and surgical nursing units
- nursery
- telemetry
- labor and delivery room
- diagnostic laboratories
- physical therapy
- recovery room
- surgery
- central supply and service
- pulmonary function
- respiratory/inhalation therapy
- blood bank
- cardiac catheterization
- discharge planning
- intensive care units
- EKG
- diagnostic radiology
- therapeutic radiology
- anesthesia
- physical medicine
- cardiac rehabilitation
- emergency room
- pharmacy

- outpatient clinics
- speech and language therapy
- social service
- occupational therapy
- EEG

## Patient Care Support

Patient care support cost centers generally provide the room, board, and recordkeeping functions for patients. They may also provide services that are ultimately consumed by another hospital cost center (for example, surgical instrument tray sterilization and wrapping). Patient care support cost centers typically include:

- dietary
- housekeeping
- admitting/registration
- central sterilization
- patient billing/cashiering
- laundry and linen
- patient transportation
- medical records
- materials distribution
- tumor registry

## General Overhead

General overhead cost centers perform centralized business functions for the institution (for example, payroll) or provide services for the convenience of the institution as a whole (for example, the cafeteria). Fluctuations in their costs are related to activities and actions that are usually independent of patient volumes. Their costs are allocated to each other, to direct patient care, and to patient care support cost centers and are recognized generally as overhead. The business functions of general overhead cost centers include:

- administration
- data processing
- payroll
- information

- personnel
- financial accounting
- general education
- collections
- public relations
- purchasing
- mailroom/receiving
- planning
- parking
- security

Other functions of general overhead cost centers include:

- engineering and plant
- cafeteria
- in-service education
- maintenance
- infection control
- employee health
- biomedical engineering

### Medical Education

Medical education cost centers are directly related to a graduate medical education (GME) program. Many teaching hospitals require that their direct GME costs be isolated when they analyze their effects on product and product-line profitability. By isolating its direct GME costs, a hospital can compare its product and product-line costs with both teaching and nonteaching hospitals in its service area and regionally and nationally. Also, third party payers in competitive bidding proposals often ask that price schedules isolate direct GME costs. In this way, some comparability among competing hospitals can be achieved. However, indirect teaching costs, such as those for additional ancillary services, should be isolated and accounted for in order to identify GME costs completely.

GME costs are generally reimbursed by some incremental amount if the teaching hospital is selected in a competitive bidding situation. Research costs can be handled either as a separate category, like that for medical education, or as a subcategory within medical education.

## Control Period Selection

The second organizational step is to select a control period to serve as the basis for gathering resource, cost, activity, and statistical information. The cost and statistical information will be used to assess the reasonableness of the cost management system's derived ("earned") results, based on procedure volumes from the control period.

An historical period rather than a budget period is preferred for control purposes, since budgeted figures generally have no solid basis for their composition (for example, adding five percent to last year's budget) and are normally not based on procedural cost data or activity volumes.

In the selection of the control (historical) period, several criteria must be met. The first is that the control period must reflect current operations and services as much as possible. In this way, historical costs, statistics, and procedure volumes will be available for most, if not all, of the cost centers and procedures. Inquiries regarding major renovations in physical plant, equipment replacements or upgrades, and the addition of new programs and services can be used to determine the appropriateness of a particular period.

The second criterion involves the integrity of the historical period's financial and statistical data. Many times, the hospital's various transaction systems will contain inaccuracies, for example, "float" personnel salaries and hours recorded in only one instead of two or three cost centers. Depending on their magnitude and frequency, these inaccuracies may severely impact the integrity of the data collected and impede the reasonableness testing process. Therefore, it is imperative that all questions regarding inaccuracies be thoroughly answered and documented during the review of transaction systems in the initial conceptual design documentation phase. If this is done, fewer surprises will surface during the implementation process.

Finally, it is preferable to use data for a full fiscal year. This generally eliminates integrity problems associated with accruals, inventory, and intermittent spending patterns (for example, legal or audit fees).

If the hospital faces severe constraints, such as new services or programs or a staggered implementation timetable, the appropriateness of alternative control periods may be investigated. This investigation should be the responsibility of the task force project director. The integrity of the alternative periods' data should be challenged, and the impact that possible inaccuracies in the data may have on the data-gathering and reasonableness testing process should be assessed. To avoid future surprises, all significant findings and an estimation of their impact on the cost management project's implementation should be communicated to the task force.

Once the control period has been selected, the following financial and statistical information should be obtained for the period:

- year-to-date general ledger expenses, by cost center and subaccount (for example, medical supplies, chemicals)
- year-to-date worked payroll hours, by cost center, skill level (for example, RN), and type (for example, vacation, holiday)
- a procedure listing (generally from the charge master), including procedure number, description, and year-to-date volume
- a fixed asset listing, by cost center, including identification (tag) number, description, and year-to-date depreciation

Supplemental *current period* data may also be collected at this time. These data come from transaction system source documents, indicating unit costs and revenue figures. They include:

- current-period average labor rates, by cost center and skill level
- current-period published procedure unit revenues
- listing of supply items (from the hospital's materials management system), including item number, description, and current period unit cost

Current, rather than control period, cost data are preferable in the case of the above items, since current costs are more up-to-date and the relevant source documents are more readily available.

The above organizational information is used as the basis to support the procedure resource and cost standards setting process (for example, procedure listing, average labor rates) while others are used as data inputs for reasonableness testing (for example, procedure volumes). A detailed discussion of how this information is used is presented in the standards setting and reasonableness testing sections of this chapter.

### Classification of General Ledger Subaccounts as Fixed or Variable

The third organizational step involves classifying each cost center's general ledger expense subaccounts as either fixed or variable. These classifications are used when summarizing the control period's costs for reasonableness testing and data-gathering purposes and when designating subaccounts for future budgeting and performance-reporting applications.

The limitations of hospital cost management and transaction systems generally preclude the classification of costs as other than fixed or variable. However, cost behavior may be affected by relevant range issues, which may require alternative classifications.

The process of determining fixed or variable cost behavior involves an analysis of how the costs that are recorded in each general ledger subaccount react according to fluctuations in cost center activity. A listing of a hospital's general ledger and cost center subaccounts can usually be obtained from the hospital's accounting personnel. General ledger expense subaccounts that typically fall under fixed and variable headings by natural expense classification are shown in Table 7–1.

## Calculation of Control Totals

The final organizational step involves totaling each cost center's control-period general ledger subaccount costs and labor hours by skill level and type, according to their fixed and variable cost designations by natural expense classifications (for example, labor, benefits, supply/ other, or capital). For example, a control total figure for rents and leases, equipment maintenance contracts, and warranty costs for each cost center is calculated, since all of these subaccount costs are fixed and fall under the capital natural expense classification. This figure is then compared with the costs calculated by the cost management system to determine the reasonableness of the standards data. Some amounts calculated in this step may also serve as inputs to cost management software systems.

Initially, the control period's total fixed supply and capital-related costs may be sufficient for the purpose of cost management system inputs. Over time, however, these data may be revised to reflect the actual or budgeted amounts of other periods.

## PROCEDURE IDENTIFICATION AND SELECTION

The objective of the procedure identification and selection process is to, first, identify each cost center's procedures based on existing documentation (for example, the hospital's charge master), and, second, to select those procedures within each cost center for which detailed resource and cost standards will be determined.

**Table 7-1** General Ledger Expense Subaccounts Classified as Fixed or Variable

| Fixed | Variable |
|---|---|
| Labor: | Labor: |
| Administrators | Staff RN |
| Managers | LPN |
| Head nurse | Aide |
| Executive secretaries | Technicians |
| Supervisors (partial) | Clerks |
| | Environmental and food workers |
| | Transporters |
| | Line secretaries |
| | Supervisors (partial) |
| Benefits: | Benefits: |
| Statutory and elective benefits defined as fixed in nature | Statutory and elective benefits in relation to variable salary |
| Pension payouts | |
| Supply/other: | Supply/other: |
| Legal and audit fees | Postage |
| Nonclinical consulting services | Professional clinical fees |
| Travel, dues, and seminars | Medical/surgical supplies |
| Cleaning supplies (partial) | Chemicals and reagents |
| Minor equipment | Cleaning supplies (partial) |
| Miscellaneous | Pharmaceuticals |
| Telephone | Oxygen and other medical gases |
| Office and general supplies | IV solutions and admin sets |
| Fuel and utilities | Prosthesis |
| Malpractice insurance | Films, solutions, and paper |
| | Whole blood |
| | Radioactive materials |
| | Purchased clinical services |
| | Food |
| | Linens and sheets |
| | Purchased food or housekeeping services |
| | Cleaning supplies |
| Capital: | Capital: |
| Depreciation | None |
| Interest | |
| Rent/lease | |
| Equipment maintenance and warranty contracts | |
| Asset insurance | |
| Property taxes | |
| License fees | |

A discussion of the procedure identification and selection approach, by cost center type, is presented in the following sections.

## Nursing Units

For nursing units, costs vary based on the patient's illness, severity, and psychosociological attributes. As a surrogate for collecting costs based on these attributes, nursing costs can be captured using a patient classification system; that is, the procedures can be represented by acuity levels within the patient classification system. Ideally, no more than five to six acuity levels per cost center should be identified as procedures, because finer distinctions generally do not vary enough in resource consumption and clinical meaningfulness. Also, by limiting the number of acuity levels to five or six, the incorporation of acuity levels into the hospital's billing system and the product resource consumption profiles is more easily accomplished and maintained.

In the case of those patient classification systems that assign patient acuity on wide-ranging point-scoring schemes, it may be necessary to collapse the point ranges into five or six acuity-range categories. These revisions should be carefully reviewed to ensure that they are consistent with the cost management system's goals and objectives (for example, resulting in a reasonable number of acuity levels).

If patients are not currently being charged by acuity level on the hospital's billing system, additional tasks will be required to incorporate patient acuity into the product resource consumption profiles. In this situation, a sampling of historical patient data will be necessary to document the number of days by acuity level and product, and that information can then be incorporated into the product's resource consumption profile.

If the hospital does not have a patient classification system, nursing procedures will equate to an "average" patient day of care. This may have to suffice in the short term, since a patient classification system usually takes four to six months to implement. However, caution should be exercised when interpreting and analyzing the costs and profitability of products (case types) using an "average" patient day of care. Studies have shown that direct nursing resources and the costs of the lowest-to-highest acuity levels may differ by more than 500 percent.

Depending on a product's related nursing requirements and length of stay, its cost and profitability may not be known until nursing acuity information is brought into the cost management system. Moreover, unless the patient acuity data are integrated into the cost management system, the full value of performance-monitoring and budgeting applications in the nursing areas will not be realized.

A patient classification system can provide hospitals with accurate nursing resource and cost information by patient, clinical documentation, and staffing optimization. Thus, if such a system does not exist, the hospital should seriously consider implementing one. Hospitals with existing patient classification systems should review them to ascertain their capabilities to meet the hospital's needs and objectives.

## Ancillary Cost Centers

Ancillary cost centers' procedures are initially identified by using the hospital's charge master. A typical charge master for a 500-bed hospital has approximately 6,000 to 10,000 ancillary charge items (procedures). The number of procedures on the charge master for each cost center can range from as few as five to as many as several thousand for pharmacy and central supply cost centers.

To reduce the number of ancillary procedures for which detailed standard costing studies will be undertaken, the "80/20 rule" should be applied to the procedures in each ancillary cost center. In this way, only those procedures that are significant in volume and cost will have detailed standards set. If detailed standard costing studies are not going to be performed for a cost center's procedures (for example, using ratio of cost-to-charge, RCC, or relative value unit, RVU, costing), an 80/20 selection process is not required.

The 80/20 selection process uses a two-pass approach. In the first pass, those procedures whose cumulative activity meets or exceeds 80 percent (or 90 percent) of the cost center's total *activity* are selected. In the second pass, those procedures whose revenue cumulatively meets or exceeds 80 percent (or 90 percent) of the cost center's total *revenue* are selected. This two-pass approach produces a listing of procedures that represents a minimum of 80 percent (or 90 percent) of the cost center's activities and variable costs.

The procedure selection process may be broadened to include some procedures that fall into the 20-percent category if they have a high unit charge (for example, over $100). The supporting argument would be that these procedures may be common to a particular product, thereby significantly influencing that product's cost.

It is generally unnecessary to perform an 80/20 analysis for ancillary cost centers that have only 25 to 30 procedures listed on the charge master. For these cost centers, it is recommended that all procedures have detailed standards set. The specific cut-off for the minimum number of procedures within a cost center that will have detailed standards set should be discussed with the task force and finalized prior to the procedure selection process.

## Patient Care Support Cost Centers

Patient care support cost centers (for example, laundry and dietary) generally have no predefined procedures. The identification of procedures in these cost centers involves the documentation of their activities and outputs. This procedure-identification documentation is part of the cost center operations documentation process (described in detail later in this chapter).

In many instances, the identification and documentation of patient care support cost center procedures are addressed as long-term objectives. In the short term, a single global procedure may be used in lieu of specific procedure identification. In this case, it is generally recommended that the costs of the patient care support departments be allocated to direct patient care cost centers, using some type of gross-output-oriented statistic, for example, meals served, pounds of laundry, etc.

If the hospital decides to develop detailed standard resource and cost profiles for the procedures and not allocate their cost centers' costs, the procedures and their respective consumption will need to be listed on each product's resource consumption profile. In the short term, a sampling of the procedures' consumption by product is the recommended basis for listing them on each product resource consumption profile. In the long term, it is best to use the hospital's billing system to document the periodic activity of each patient support procedure and the consumption of the procedures by product. In this way, a single hospital transaction system can capture the procedure activity and consumption data, eliminating the need for sampling and possible multiple transaction system interfaces.

## General Overhead and Medical Education

General overhead and medical education cost centers generally employ the same procedure identification and selection process that patient care support cost centers employ. Over the long term, it is recommended that specific procedures be identified and standard resource and cost profiles be developed to bring these cost centers into the hospital's cost management system's performance reporting and budgeting applications. However, once identified, it is unnecessary to integrate the procedures into the product resource consumption profiles. Rather they should be used solely for budgeting and intra-cost-center performance evaluation purposes.

For example, the resources and costs of a hospital's maintenance cost center vary with the number and magnitude of work orders, which are independent of patient activity fluctuations. The work orders reflect the manpower and supply requirements to renovate the physical plant or to preserve the existing condition of equipment. By identifying the type of work orders (for example, 80–100 manhours, 101–120 manhours, etc.) and forecasting the volume of each, the hospital is able to budget maintenance cost center resource and cost requirements more accurately.

By extending the actual volume for each type of work order performed during a reporting period against standard costs, an "earned" budget can be calculated for the maintenance cost center. This earned budget can then be compared with actual resource and cost consumption to assess the efficiency of the maintenance cost center in meeting its workload demand.

### Procedure Listing

Once procedures are identified from existing documentation and the selection of the procedures to be detail-costed is completed (for example, by an 80/20 analysis), two procedure lists should be developed for each cost center. The first list will show those procedures for which detailed costing studies will be performed (a listing of 80/20 procedures). The second list will show those procedures to be costed by using less sophisticated techniques. Each list should indicate each procedure's number and provide a narrative description of the procedure. (A detailed discussion on procedure costing techniques is presented in a later section in this chapter.)

## COST CENTER OPERATIONS DOCUMENTATION

The next major task to be performed is to document each cost center's operations. This is an important step toward understanding fully the functions and activities of a cost center and its unique production problems. In addition, the deficiencies in the hospital transaction systems as they may affect a particular cost center should be documented. Figure 7–2 depicts the objectives and results of the operations documentation process.

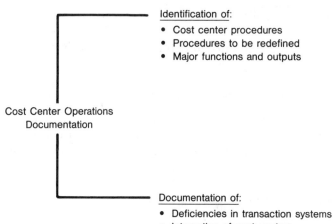

Identification of:
- Cost center procedures
- Procedures to be redefined
- Major functions and outputs

Cost Center Operations
Documentation

Documentation of:
- Deficiencies in transaction systems
- Interaction of cost centers
- General flow and capacity issues

**Figure 7–2** Operations Documentation Outputs

## Method

The best way to carry out the documentation task is to develop a cost center documentation questionnaire. This questionnaire should cover such issues as:

- how the cost center is organized
- whether outside services are used to perform procedures
- what the cost center's minimum staffing requirements and current production capacity estimates are
- what services are provided for and by other cost centers, and how they are recorded on the hospital's transaction systems
- which procedures with a single charge number incur a different resource intensity, and how that intensity should be weighed, based on historical workloads
- how procedures are scheduled and the scheduling problems that might occur
- how supplies are recorded on financial records (expensed, inventoried, spoiled)
- what the deficiencies in working conditions are, such as improper physical layout and outdated automation

**Outcome**

The operations documentation process should achieve the following results.

*Identification of Cost Center Procedures*

The identification of a cost center's procedures is particularly important in the case of overhead and patient care support cost centers that generally do not have a predefined listing of procedures. The resulting information may then be used by the hospital to set standards for all cost centers, in order to facilitate performance reporting and budgeting applications and refine patient resource consumption by product.

*Redefinition of Existing Procedures*

The process should serve to identify existing procedures that may need to be redefined into a series of procedures, in order to account properly for significant resource and cost intensity differences (for example, based on patient condition, the location where the procedure is performed, or the fact that the procedure is required on an immediate or stat basis). In the short term, the resulting information can be used to weight a procedure's resources and costs, based on the extension of fluctuation in its resource requirements (for example, 15 minutes of labor time, 30 minutes of labor time), by the frequency of their occurrence (for example, 15 minutes of labor time required by 20 percent of the patients). In the long term, if these differences are significant in amount and frequency of occurrence, it is better to account for them as separate procedures. This is generally accomplished by establishing unique procedure descriptions and numbers that reflect the differences in resources (for example, EKG 15–30 minutes, EKG 31–45 minutes, etc.). Changes in the hospital's procedure recording system (for example, the charge system) must be coordinated with the fiscal and data-processing managers and the initiating cost center's manager to determine if data-processing constraints exist.

The benefit of revising procedure definitions due to resource and cost differences is threefold:

1. The procedures are more definitive as to the resources required to perform them for a particular patient and thus may further document the condition of a patient, for example, severity of illness.
2. If the differences in resource requirements for an individual procedure are accounted for through the use of multiple procedure

descriptions, efficiency analyses and cost center workload budget demands are more easily calculated, due to the elimination of averaging techniques.

3. Calculation of the cost of products is more accurate, since the cost of the procedures are not represented by broad averages (for example, encompassing labor requirements ranging from 15 to 120 minutes or supply costs ranging from $5 to $100). This can enhance the profitability and margin analysis of products, product lines, and physicians.

## Identification of Major Functions and Outputs

The operations documentation process serves to identify major functions and outputs (for example, patient assessments and special dietary consultations) that are not recorded on any existing hospital system and whose absence will adversely affect patient resource consumption documentation and the cost center's performance evaluation reporting. These functions and outputs may be added to the cost center's 80/20 procedure listing as a basis for developing its resource and cost profiles for the short term. In this case, a mechanism to record their periodic activity and product consumption needs to be implemented. For this purpose, a manual recording system is generally used.

In the long term, these functions and outputs are normally put into the hospital's charge master to facilitate volume and product consumption recordkeeping. By recognizing and recording these activities in this way, their impact on treatment protocols (for example, special dietary consultation to reduce the length of stay) can be documented, thereby improving treatment protocols and reducing costs.

## Confirmation of Deficiencies

The operations documentation process can confirm deficiencies in hospitalwide transaction systems (for example, payroll, general ledger) that specifically affect a cost center (for example, by improperly recording "float" or cross-trained personnel time or by expensing supplies rather than inventorying them) and the magnitude of the deficiency. In this case, the documentation serves two purposes. First, it may explain why there are differences between system-derived "earned" resource and cost data and control period resource and cost data during reasonableness testing. Second, it may confirm transaction system deficiencies and their magnitude with regard to individual cost centers, possibly signifying a need to replace an existing transaction system.

*Indication of Cost Center Interaction*

The operations documentation process reveals the interaction of cost centers (for example, central sterilization providing services to the surgery cost center, the sharing of common equipment) and shows how the scheduling and recording of services between cost centers is handled. This can highlight possible coordination problems between cost centers that may interrupt the patient-treatment or supply-procurement process.

*Existence of Flow and Capacity Issues*

Finally, the operations documentation process can pinpoint general flow and capacity issues, such as:

- physical layout inadequacies
- scheduling/communication problems
- equipment inadequacies
- significant changes in operation (for example, elimination of services, new services, new equipment)
- inefficiencies due to low-quality supplies

The documentation of flow and capacity problems may explain why a cost center operates inefficiently. Once the problems are documented, solutions can be formulated, generally resulting in decreased costs and higher quality and profitability.

**Related Issues**

The process of completing the cost center operations documentation questionnaire involves meeting with the cost center manager to discuss each question and to document responses. Experience has shown that, when cost center managers are asked to complete the questionnaire independently, they usually produce incomplete or vague responses, for example, by not attaching requested support documentation or by failing to identify specific procedures that need to be redefined.

Practice has shown that the problems arising in the cost center operations documentation process can be grouped into three major categories:

1. organizational issues
2. procedure definition issues
3. standard resource and cost determination issues

## Organizational Issues

A typical organizational issue concerns the managerial responsibility for multiple cost centers. For example, a single manager might be responsible for both the EKG and EEG cost centers of the hospital. The manager might spend 35 percent of available time on EKG-related activities and 65 percent on EEG-related activities. However, in the hospital's payroll and general ledger systems, all of the manager's time and related expenses are recorded and reported in the EEG cost center. No transfer of these hours and expenses are ever made to the EKG cost center. Resources and costs (labor, supplies, and equipment) that are used in the performance of EKG and EEG procedures are appropriately accounted for and properly recorded in their respective cost centers.

One possible solution to this problem is to establish a separate and distinct cost center to account for and record those resources and costs that are incurred only by, and are attributable solely to, the managerial activities of multiple cost centers. By using this approach, the forecasting and monitoring of resources in all cost centers can be improved since resources and costs are segregated and associated with their true activities and functions. The new cost center would then be classified as an overhead cost center and its costs allocated to the user cost centers on some rational basis (for example, time spent, FTEs, etc.).

## Procedure Definition Issues

A typical procedure definition issue results when different supplies are used for the same procedure. For example, in a cardiac catheterization department, there may be a single charge number for the heart catheterization procedure. This is because labor time and personnel mix is virtually identical for all catheterizations. However, the major supply item, catheters, for the heart catheterization procedure can be any one of 20 catheters, ranging in price from $5 to $118. Moreover, the same catheter is used in about 90 percent of all heart catheterization procedures.

One option to clarify this situation may be to set up unique charge numbers for each major supply item (for example, the catheter). The common labor and minor supply items would then be accounted for under a separate charge number, independently of that used for the catheter. This approach would greatly enhance the hospital's ability to determine, monitor, and forecast the use of catheters and catheter costs.

Another option may be to use a unique charge number for the catheterizations that use the same catheter 90 percent of the time. The charge number would cover all relevant resources (for example, labor, catheter, common minor supplies, and equipment resources). For the catheterizations that use any one of the other 19 catheters, another unique charge number would be used. This charge number could again cover all relevant resources. The cost of the catheter components would be accounted for by using a weighted average of their costs, based on a sampling of their usage.

### Standard Resource and Cost Determination Issues

One of the difficult questions regarding standard resource and cost setting issues is how to account for minimum staffing. One alternative is to record all minimum staffing hours as a fixed component in the cost management system. By adopting this approach, management recognizes that a certain level of staffing is required regardless of activity, possibly due to legal, accreditation, or philosophical reasons. The drawback of the approach is manifested when the same staff personnel actually produce procedures, thereby causing a double counting of their time.

For example, assume that on the third shift minimum staffing personnel actually produce procedures that require 3 hours of production time and that there are 8 available shift hours. In this situation the cost management system would record 8 hours (fixed) of minimum staffing and 3 direct production hours, for a total of 11 hours required for the minimum staffing personnel for that shift, indicating a productivity rate of 137 percent. If there were no activity at all for the cost center for a given period of time, the cost management system would show no variance between required and staffed hours, even though actual productivity was zero, thereby masking a potentially serious problem.

An alternative solution would be to decide that no minimum staffing hours would be recorded as a fixed component in the cost management system. By adopting this approach, management implicitly assumes that all production people within the cost center should be productive to justify their existence. The drawback of this approach is manifested when the minimum staffing personnel are not utilized fully, producing a continuing variance in the system.

For example, suppose that a minimum staffing individual on the third shift actually produced procedures that required 6 hours of production time, out of a total of 8 available shift hours. The cost management system would record a total of 6 required hours for this individual for that shift, or a productivity rate of 75 percent. The system also would report an unfavorable variance of 2 hours from actual staffing. If there were no activity in the department for a period of time, the required productivity rate would be zero, while actual staffing would be 8 hours, thereby causing an unfavorable variance of 8 hours and highlighting a potential problem.

Regardless of the method selected to record minimum staffing, although it should be consistent for all cost centers, the staffing should be identified by shift and by person (name) for each cost center. Discussions with cost center personnel can facilitate this process.

**Follow-Up**

All significant issues identified during the cost center operations documentation process that may affect data integrity or impede the data-gathering process should be summarized and communicated to the task force. The task force should then act on each issue and resolve it to the satisfaction of all parties. In this process, short-term and long-term solutions are usually developed to prevent delaying the implementation of the cost management system. In some cases, if an issue is common to many cost centers and is of significant importance, the project may have to be delayed.

**SELECTING A STANDARD-SETTING METHODOLOGY**

The next step in the procedure standard development process involves the selection of a methodology to gather the requisite resource and cost standards data for those procedures selected for detailed standard costing. In addition, a methodology to determine the standards for a cost center's residual procedures (those in the 20-percent group) must be selected.

**Methodologies for 80/20 Procedures**

Various methodologies are available to develop procedural resource and cost standards for 80/20 procedures. The most common methodologies are:

- technical estimates
- industrial engineering techniques
- predetermined standards

In the following sections, each of these methodologies is described and the costs and benefits associated with each methodology are listed and compared.

### Technical Estimates

Technical estimates constitute a common short-term methodology for determining the standard resource consumption and cost of a particular procedure. Technical estimates require that a specialist identify and document the types and quantities of resources expected to be consumed by a specific procedure during its normal production cycle. The estimates are based on the specialist's knowledge of a particular cost center's functions, understanding how the estimates will ultimately be used, and familiarity with the cost center's production process (for example, physical layout, scheduling, automation, etc.). Labor, material, and equipment resource items, with their related procedure usage and unit costs, are identified and documented in a walk-through of each procedure's production process. Group discussions and consultations with technical personnel should augment the standard-setting process when necessary. If the process is properly completed, only a single estimate will be needed. Generally, the hospital's cost center managers and their technical personnel are responsible for developing the technical estimates.

The technical-estimates methodology is recommended for initially developing procedural resource and cost standards because it provides these advantages:

- It can be applied in nearly every cost center (generally, the exception is nursing).
- It can be implemented with a minimal amount of training.
- As shown in management engineering research studies, its results may be 80 to 85 percent as accurate as engineered standards.
- It permits hospital specialists (for example, clinical managers) to be recommended and used to perform the resource identification and documentation tasks, thereby reducing project costs.
- It generally does not interfere with the normal work routine of the cost center.

- It documents all types of resources, not just labor.
- Because the hospital managers have helped to develop them, its resulting standards are more likely to be accepted at the managerial level.
- Its standards can be developed across departments typically within three months.

The following are some of the disadvantages of the technical-estimates methodology:

- The documentation may not always be complete. For example, supply descriptions may be missing.
- Cost center managers may overestimate labor requirements to provide a "safety cushion."
- There is no evaluation of best methods (for example, regarding system improvements) before the estimates are made. This means that resources and costs are based on previous knowledge, and the hospital postpones the opportunity to identify opportunities to cut costs.

## Industrial Engineering Techniques

Throughout the years, a variety of industrial engineering techniques have been developed to enable management to estimate work in terms of a standard. The most common of these techniques are time-and-motion studies, work sampling, and self-logging.

**Time-and-Motion Studies.** A common method used to measure work (particularly in manufacturing organizations) is the time-and-motion study. This method divides the operation to be studied into elements, each of which is timed with a stopwatch. Because of delay factors involved and the relative complexity of many tasks, it is common practice to divide tasks into specific elements. These elements are usually groups of basic motion and are long enough (usually one-half minute) to be practical. The number of timings required is determined statistically, by the amount of variation, the proportion of the element to the whole, and the final use of the time.

There are several advantages in the use of this technique:

- It provides an accurate measurement of time (acceptable to management and cost center managers).

- It often includes an evaluation of the activities performed and efforts to improve them before the standards are set (in contrast to the a priori nature of technical estimates).
- It permits allowances for personal, fatigue, and delay (PFD) time to be incorporated into the standards.

However, time-and-motion studies have distinct disadvantages as well:

- The development of time-and-motion standards is extremely time-intensive.
- Stopwatch timing can create a morale problem if not properly presented to employees.
- The stopwatch is generally unsatisfactory for measuring long-cycle activities or work that is varied in nature (the latter in particular is a problem in health care).
- Trained personnel are needed to perform the study.
- The analysis of time logs may be costly and time-consuming because of the volume of paper produced.

**Work Sampling.** Another common method of work measurement is work sampling. This is a statistical technique for analyzing activity times. It is based on the laws of probability and operates on the premise that a random sample drawn from a large group will tend to resemble that group. The larger the sample size, the more confidence there will be in the times determined.

The technique requires observations to be made at random times throughout the working day. Note that the random sample is not a haphazard selection; it is obtained by ensuring that each item has an identical chance of being selected. Thus, both the observation times and the sequences must be determined randomly. In applying this technique to work measurement, the percentage of the work day spent in each of the various activities and the percentage of time the worker is idle or away from the work area are determined. An example of a work-sampling form is shown as Exhibit 7–1.

The key factor in the success of a work-sampling measurement study is accuracy in determining and obtaining the proper number of observations. Once the percentage occurrence of the activity under study has been estimated and the desired accuracy of the sample has been stated, the specific number of random samples that are needed can be determined mathematically.

Work sampling offers a number of advantages:

- It is relatively inexpensive to apply (compared with time-and-motion studies).
- It does not interfere with the normal routine of the cost center.
- It can be done without lengthy technical training.
- It produces results that are known to be reliable and accurate.

The following are some of the disadvantages of work sampling:

- It does not provide a detailed record of the conditions under which the work is performed.
- It does not permit an easy classification of the work into detailed procedures; rather it categorizes the work in major work activities.
- It does permit the capture of data on supply and equipment resource use.
- It is an a priori measurement of current practice.

**Self-Logging.** Another work measurement technique is self-logging. This is a participative work measurement technique by which employees record their own time and volume data. With this technique, each employee maintains a daily log of activities or a record of log-in/log-out activities. The activities to be measured are determined and described in advance. After the logs have been kept for a statistically defined period of time, the accumulated time and volume data are summarized and averaged to determine the time required per activity.

The advantages of self-logging are several:

- It is easy to implement.
- It is easy to understand and is acceptable to employees.
- It does not require elaborate training to be applied.

The following are disadvantages to self-logging:

- Close monitoring is required (carelessness in recording times and volumes may produce errors).
- Although time logs are simple to install, their analysis may be costly and time-consuming because of the volume of paper produced.

**Exhibit 7–1** Example of a Work-Sampling Form

Date _____

| PERSONNEL NAME/TYPE OF PERSONNEL | 7:00 | 7:15 | 7:30 | 7:45 | 8:00 | 8:15 | 8:30 | 8:45 | 9:00 | 9:15 | 9:30 | 9:45 | 10:00 | 10:15 | 10:30 |
|---|---|---|---|---|---|---|---|---|---|---|---|---|---|---|---|
| | | | | | | | | | | | | | | | |
| | | | | | | | | | | | | | | | |
| | | | | | | | | | | | | | | | |
| | | | | | | | | | | | | | | | |
| | | | | | | | | | | | | | | | |
| | | | | | | | | | | | | | | | |
| | | | | | | | | | | | | | | | |
| | | | | | | | | | | | | | | | |
| | | | | | | | | | | | | | | | |
| | | | | | | | | | | | | | | | |
| | | | | | | | | | | | | | | | |
| | | | | | | | | | | | | | | | |
| | | | | | | | | | | | | | | | |
| | | | | | | | | | | | | | | | |
| | | | | | | | | | | | | | | | |
| | | | | | | | | | | | | | | | |
| | | | | | | | | | | | | | | | |
| | | | | | | | | | | | | | | | |
| | | | | | | | | | | | | | | | |
| | | | | | | | | | | | | | | | |
| | | | | | | | | | | | | | | | |

TIME OF OBSERVATION

## OBSERVATION CODE

*Activity*

| | | | |
|---|---|---|---|
| D | - Direct Patient Care | OI | - Other Indirect Care |
| DO | - Direct Patient Care Off Dept. | SB | - Stand-By |
| T | - Transport Patient | PT | - Personal Time |
| MP | - Meet with Physician | DC | - Documentation |
| S | - Staff/Student Supervision | PC | - Phone Calls |
| FC | - Family Conferences | C | - Clerical |
| RM | - Rehab Staffing Meeting | SH | - Scheduling |
| SM | - Staff Meeting/In Service | P | - Patient Conference |
| TT | - Teaching/Training | | (Rounds/Rehab Staff/ |
| HC | - Housekeeping/Cleaning | | Family Contracts) |

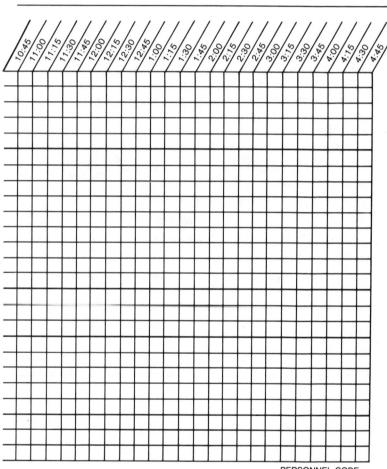

PERSONNEL CODE

01 - Therapist
02 - P.T. Assistant
03 - Transporter
04 - Aide
05 - Secretary
06 - Director

- Data on supply and equipment resource usage are generally not captured.
- Self-logging is an a priori measurement.

## Predetermined Standards

Predetermined standards may be used in lieu of standard-setting methodologies that are hospital-specific participative or observation-oriented. Predetermined standards are management-engineered standards (using the above-defined techniques) that apply across a representative sample of hospitals. For hospital-specific use, however, the standards have to be challenged and evaluated against the hospital's particular operations.

There are several advantages to the use of predetermined standards:

- They provide an impartial time standard (valid across institutions).
- They are relatively inexpensive to implement.
- Compared with other methodologies, they are the least disruptive to current operations.
- Their maintenance costs are low and changes are easily made.
- They are usually based on time-and-motion studies over a range of hospitals.
- They do not include current operating inefficiencies.

The following are some disadvantages to the use of predetermined standards:

- Resistance to their use for performance monitoring may arise if the cost center manager has no input to ensure their reasonableness.
- Supply and equipment resource type and usage are usually not considered when setting the standards.
- Such factors as working conditions, automation, and employee training must be noted and verified.
- They are generally not available for all cost centers.
- Generally, no detail is available to promote budgeting and performance monitoring at a skill or general ledger level.
- They may need to be customized for differences between hospital areas.

*Summary*

Any of the above methodologies can be used to measure resource consumption for a particular 80/20 procedure. That is, each can be used to determine the time and supplies required to perform a particular job. There is no universally best methodology to use for 80/20 procedures. The best technique for a particular situation will depend on the time available, the relevant budget and manpower constraints, and the end use of the data.

Due to the level of detail generally required by a cost management system and the relatively low cost involved, most hospitals use the technical-estimates and the predetermined-standards methodologies as the initial means to set 80/20 procedure resource and cost standards. If hospitals wish to update their standards, one or several of the industrial engineering techniques can be used.

Based on our classification of hospitals, recommended resource and cost standard-setting methodologies for 80/20 procedures are presented in Table 7–2.

## Methodologies for Non-80/20 Procedures

There are several methodologies that may be considered for determining resource consumption of a cost center's procedures that are not selected for detailed costing studies. These include:

- cross-mapping
- the use of available industry RVUs
- the use of cost-to-charge ratios to convert labor and supply dollar values

**Table 7–2** Recommended Resource and Cost Standard-Setting Methodologies for 80/20 Procedures

| Hospital Type | Short-Term Methodology | Long-Term Methodology |
| --- | --- | --- |
| Small to medium | Technical estimates | Predetermined standards |
| Medium to large | Predetermined standards/ technical estimates | Industrial engineered standards |

*Cross-Mapping*

Cross-mapping procedures require the attachment of a detail-costed (80/20) procedure's resources and costs to a nondetailed costed (non-80/20) procedure. In effect, the resources and costs of the former become the surrogate resources and costs of the latter. The information required to perform this process is obtained from a matrix that lists 80/20 procedures under one heading and non-80/20 procedures under another. The initial matrix generally takes one to four hours to be prepared, per cost center, by clerical personnel. The cost center manager completes the matrix by identifying the resources of an 80/20 procedure that most closely approximate the resources of a particular non-80/20 procedure.

For example, assume that a wrist x-ray procedure was selected for detailed costing and that an ankle x-ray procedure was not; the wrist procedure is an 80/20 procedure, whereas the ankle procedure falls into the 20-percent group. If the cost center manager concludes that the ankle procedure's resources are comparable with those of the wrist procedure, the latter's resources and costs become the resources and costs of the ankle procedure.

A mapping of various procedures, one for labor and one for supply resources, may be done to refine this process. The mapping process generally requires one to three hours of a cost center manager's time.

The following are advantages of cross-mapping:

- All resources and costs are hospital-specific.
- Detail (for example, skill levels) are recognized for all procedures.
- Cost center managers have input into the process.
- Both labor and supply usage data are captured.

The major disadvantage of cross-mapping is that it requires monitoring and follow-up to ensure it meets predetermined deadlines.

*Industry RVUs*

The use of industry standards requires an available outside source (for example, a hospital association). When the standards become available, the hospital's non-80/20 procedure descriptions are matched to the standards' descriptions, thereby assigning RVU values. These RVU values are then converted to hospital-specific resource and cost values. This is done by dividing selected 80/20-procedure resources and costs (derived from technical estimates or engineering studies) by their RVU values. This produces an RVU conversion factor that can then be applied to non-80/20 procedures.

For example, assume that a chest x-ray procedure was selected for detailed costing and that a hip x-ray procedure was not (again, the chest procedure is an 80/20 procedure, while the hip falls into the 20 percent group). Further assume that each chest x-ray requires 40 minutes of direct labor and $8 of direct supplies. If the chest x-ray has an RVU value of 8, each RVU point has a labor time value of 5 minutes (40 minutes divided by 8) and a supply dollar value of $1 ($8 divided by 8 RVUs). If the hip x-ray has an RVU value of 12, its labor resources are 60 minutes (5 minutes per RVU multiplied by 12), and its supply costs are $12 ($1 per RVU multiplied by 12). Generally, two to three hours of cost center manager time is required to match descriptions. The required RVU conversion calculations generally take one-half hour of clerical time.

There are these major advantages to the use of industry RVUs:

- They provide an independent measure of resource consumption.
- Their maintenance costs are low and changes are easily made.

But there are also disadvantages to the use of industry RVUs:

- Descriptions may be difficult to match.
- RVUs may not be available for all cost centers.
- Resistance to predetermined standards for performance monitoring may occur.
- Such factors as working conditions, automation, and employee training may invalidate the results of the process.

*Cost-to-Charge Ratios*

As a methodology, the use of cost-to-charge ratios is very similar to the use of industry RVUs. That is, the cost-to-charge ratios of labor time and supply costs are calculated and used as a means of assigning resources and costs to non-80/20 procedures. The only difference is that charges, instead of RVUs, are used as the weighting basis.

For example, assume that a chest x-ray procedure was selected for detailed costing and that a bone-age procedure was not (again, the chest x-ray is an 80/20 procedure, while the bone-age procedure falls into the 20 percent group). Further assume that each chest x-ray requires 40 minutes and $8 of direct supplies and that its unit revenue is $80. Therefore, each dollar of revenue equates to one-half minute of labor

(40 minutes divided by $80) and $.10 of supplies ($8 divided by $80). If the bone-age procedure's unit revenue is $100, its labor resources are 50 minutes (one-half minute of labor per revenue dollar times $100) and $10 of supplies ($.10 of supply cost per revenue dollar times $100).

These calculations are easy to perform and not very time-consuming. The major advantages of this methodology are that:

- It requires a minimal effort to understand and apply.
- Its maintenance costs are relatively low.

However, there are some distinct disadvantages to the methodology as well:

- Charges generally have no correlation with resource and cost intensity.
- There is no involvement by cost center managers.

*Summary*

Any of the above methodologies can be used to determine the resources and cost standards of non-80/20 procedures. Again, there is no universally best methodology to use; the selection will depend on the time available, the relevant economic constraints, and the intended end use of the data.

However, considering the level of detail required, and keeping in mind cost factors and the need to involve cost center managers, we recommend cross-mapping as an appropriate means of determining non-80/20 procedure resource and cost standards.

Once the residual procedure resource and cost standards are determined, the resulting information, along with each procedure's historical volumes, is formatted and entered into the cost management software program. Edit and procedure-costing reports are then produced to verify the accuracy and presence of inputs and as a basis for reviewing each procedure's direct cost profile.

## THE DATA COLLECTION PROCESS

In this section, we describe the steps involved in collecting the standard data required to implement a cost management system. These specific categories of the data collection process are discussed:

- direct procedural resource and cost standard setting (using the technical-estimates methodology previously described) and indirect cost center resource and cost standard setting
- entering the data into the cost management system
- gathering cost allocation data

## Standard Setting for Direct Procedural and Indirect Cost Center Resources and Costs

The data collection approach using direct procedural resource and cost standards as presented here is based on the use of the technical-estimate methodology described earlier. The tasks involve:

- developing a data-collection timetable
- developing data-collection worksheets
- collecting the data

### *Developing the Timetable*

A master timetable must be developed to schedule and monitor the distribution and completion of the data-collection worksheets. The basis of this timetable is a cost center and cost center manager listing. When developing the timetable, two key points need to be considered:

1. Caution should be exercised in scheduling data collection in areas that are undergoing major renovations, equipment installations, or other significant production changes. In these situations, discussions with the relevant cost center managers and their supervisors are needed to establish a practical data-collection timetable. Also, delays in data collection may be warranted because of significant changes in production (and cost) caused by technological or environmental changes.
2. The time required by cost center managers to complete the data-gathering process will vary, depending on the number of procedures to be costed, the heterogeneity of the procedures, and the overall complexity of the procedure-production process. Experience has shown that 20 to 100 hours are generally required by cost center managers to do their procedure profile resource and cost data gathering, using the technical-estimate methodology. Therefore, deadlines need to be established that are reasonable and

attainable. Once formulated, the timetable should be submitted to the task force for its comments and approval.

*Developing the Worksheets*

The second major data-collection task is to develop a series of worksheets to capture the required resource and cost data for labor, materials, and equipment. The design of the worksheets should enable them to:

- capture the appropriate level of detail required by the cost management system
- capture resource item descriptors (for example, general ledger subaccount number, supply number, etc.) to promote integration with existing transaction systems and to simplify maintenance
- be compatible with the cost management computer software's data input screens and parameters, thereby avoiding excessive data manipulations and permitting easier data entry

The task force project director should take the lead in developing the data-collection worksheets. Managers from several major cost centers (for example, surgery and radiology) also should be involved in the worksheet design process to assess the worksheets' clarity and functionality. Copies of the recommended worksheets should then be distributed to the task force members for their comments and approval.

A data-collection packet containing all worksheets and applicable source/support documents should be assembled for those cost centers that have to estimate procedure resource and cost standards. The data-collection packet should include the following seven elements:

1. an introductory/explanatory section, including a timetable
2. a listing of those procedures for which detailed standards will be set
3. a listing of those procedures that will be costed, using other costing methodologies
4. worksheets to record procedure resource and unit cost identification and documentation on labor, supplies, and equipment (including completed examples)
5. indirect resource and cost documentation worksheets on labor and supply/other costs (including completed examples)
6. the following source/support documents:

- a position control listing of each cost center's personnel
- a listing of supply items received through the central storeroom or materials management system
- a fixed asset listing
- a listing of general ledger expense subaccounts, numbers, and titles

7. a library of educational materials, including:

- a glossary of terms
- data-collection guidelines (for example, common procedure costing issues, questions, and solutions)

To expedite the data-collection process, the general information required on each worksheet (cost center name and number, procedure name and number, etc.) should be completed before the data-collection packets are distributed. This enables the cost center managers to concentrate on the documentation of procedural resource and cost data, not on clerical activities. A clerical person from the hospital's finance or accounting area is a logical choice for transcribing the general information.

Before the data-collection packets are distributed, an information and education session for the cost center managers should be conducted. The objectives of this session are to explain why the hospital is implementing a cost management system and to outline data collection responsibilities. The presentation should focus on the following issues:

- cost management concepts
- the value of a cost management system
- the methodology involved
- responsibilities for and the timetable of the data-collection process
- persons to contact for support and aid in resolving problems

In addition, the presentation should reinforce the hospital's commitment to the project and underscore the cooperation that will be expected from the audience.

As an alternative to a single presentation with all cost center managers attending, several presentations may be made for various cost center managers, keyed to their individual administrative or product-line responsibilities. In this way, more pointed discussions on responsibilities can be conducted. In practice, both single and multiple presentations have been done with equal success.

## Collecting the Data

After the timetable and the data-collection worksheets are prepared, the standards data collection process can begin. When using the technical-estimate costing methodology, two types of information must be identified and documented by cost center managers:

1. procedural resources and resource unit costs
2. cost center indirect resources and costs

To start the data collection process, meetings are scheduled with cost center managers. At these meetings, the worksheets and supporting materials of the data-collection packet are distributed and reviewed. The objective is to provide specific guidelines on what needs to be accomplished, to identify the critical deadlines, and to show how to use the worksheets and supporting documents.

For procedural resource and resource unit cost data, each of the worksheets for collecting specific components (labor, supplies, and equipment) is reviewed in detail with the relevant cost center manager. This review should include completed examples, delineating the level of detail and completeness. Supporting documents should be noted in conjunction with the worksheets, to show how they are used for documentation and reference purposes (for example, a supply listing that provides key descriptor and unit cost information).

Normally, the cost center manager should initially document resources and costs for only two or three procedures. Once that is done, a follow-up meeting can be scheduled with the manager to review the completeness and clerical accuracy of each procedure's worksheets. In this way, misinterpretations and data gathering errors can be discovered and corrected before they systematically pervade all procedures. After checking the worksheets and resolving all problems with the cost center manager, the latter should complete worksheets for the remainder of the procedures within the predefined time frame.

Next, to document indirect resources and costs, the cost center manager completes the worksheets in the cost documentation packet that address indirect labor, supplies, and capital-related resources and costs. The same interactive process previously described for procedure costing is used to review the indirect resource and cost data-collection forms and supporting documentation.

To complete the standard-setting process, a factor for personal, fatigue, and delay (PFD) time must be added to each procedure's labor standards. Though PFD varies among cost centers, it generally averages 13 to 15 percent. PFD factors may be refined through validation studies (for example, work sampling), if desired. Many software programs can adjust labor standards globally, making the incorporation of PFD factors an easy process to perform and update.

When these tasks are completed, the cost center manager should insert all relevant worksheets back into the data-collection packet and return it to the task force project director. The worksheets are then reviewed for completeness and clerical accuracy. Incomplete worksheets or worksheets that contain inaccurate data must be completed or corrected at this time to avoid inadequacies and mistakes in results and future maintenance/interface problems.

## Entering the Data into the System

After all the required data have been properly recorded, the data are formatted (if necessary) and entered into the cost management computer system. The specific data elements that are entered into the system at this point are:

- procedure descriptive information (name, number, etc.)
- procedure volumes and unit charges
- procedure direct resources and unit costs (labor, supplies, equipment)
- cost center indirect resources and costs (labor, supply/other, equipment)

After data entry is completed for a cost center, the cost management software produces two types of reports:

1. edit reports
2. procedure resource and cost reports

Edit reports are used to verify the accuracy and existence of the inputted data elements. The procedure resource and cost reports are used to confirm that the cost management system is performing the required calculations properly.

**Gathering Cost Allocation Data**

To calculate fully absorbed standard procedure costs, several types of costs have to be allocated. This requires certain algorithms and statistics. Cost allocation is a two-step process:

1. the allocation of selected cost center costs (for example, general overhead) to other cost centers
2. the allocation of cost center indirect and allocated (for example, allocated general overhead) costs to procedures

*Allocation of Selected Cost Center Costs*

The gathering of the allocation data begins by reviewing the cost centers whose costs need to be allocated. Usually these are the general overhead and medical education cost centers. In the short term, until their procedures can be identified and placed into a product's resource consumption profile, the costs of patient care support cost centers (dietary, laundry) may also be allocated.

Next, existing allocation bases and statistics are reviewed to ascertain their accuracy for the purpose of allocating costs. The Medicare cost report is generally the initial source of existing allocation data. New statistical bases are defined and new statistics developed if it is determined that the existing bases and statistics will improperly allocate costs. Existing data should be reviewed and the requisite methodologies should be developed to capture new statistical information. A list of possible allocation bases by cost center is presented in Table 7–3.

Once developed, the allocation data are formatted and entered into the cost management software program. Economies in developing and maintaining allocation statistics can be achieved by grouping all business-function cost center costs into a single amount for allocation purposes. The supporting rationale is that business functions exist for the benefit of and use by all cost centers; therefore, a single statistic can be used to allocate their costs.

The statistic that generally provides the fairest and least controversial allocation basis and thus is generally recommended for allocating the costs of business-function cost centers is gross direct costs. These cost centers can also be subdivided and allocated based on individual cost behavior (for example, labor costs for personnel). This requires a hospital decision, based on individual needs, available time and resources, and perceived level of control.

**Table 7–3** Allocation Bases by Cost Center

| Department/Cost Center Name | Allocation Basis |
|---|---|
| Accounting | |
| • Payroll function | Combine with personnel |
| • Remainder | Combine with administration |
| Administration | |
| • Building insurance | Combine with building depreciation |
| • Remainder | Accumulated direct cost |
| Audiovisual | Combine with administration |
| Biomedical engineering | Number of requisitions |
| Business office | Cost-center statistics (e.g., patient days, treatments and procedures) |
| Cafeteria | Per employee |
| Central sterilization | Time spent |
| Communications and information | |
| • Repairs and maintenance | Actual dollar amount incurred by cost center |
| • Long-distance charges | Actual dollars or a sampling of bills |
| Community relations | Combine with administration |
| Credit and collection | Combine with business office |
| Data processing | Sample of services provided to each cost center |
| Depreciation—Building | Specifically identify depreciation by individual building; allocate to cost centers based on respective square feet |
| Depreciation—Equipment | Actual by cost center, per fixed asset records |
| Dietary | Assign portion of shared salaries to cafeteria; remainder of expenses by patient days |
| Employee health | Per hour or per number of employees |
| Fiscal services | Combine with administration |
| Fringe benefits—Other | |
| • Health and dental insurance | Sample of benefits by cost center and employee; or by employee |
| • Life insurance and disability | Per employee |
| • Vacation accrual | Actual by cost center |
| Health science library | FTEs of techs and specialists, RNs and resident's accounts |

## Table 7–3 continued

| Department/Cost Center Name | Allocation Basis |
| --- | --- |
| Hospital education | Number of directors, managers, and supervisors |
| Interest expense—Building | Allocate to buildings based on original cost of buildings in mortgage; then spread to cost centers based on each cost center's square feet |
| Interest expense—Equipment | Interest from capitalized leases directly assigned to equipment covered within the lease |
| Interest expense—Operations | Combine with administration |
| Laundry | |
| • Bedding supplies | Weighted patient days (for example, medical vs. surgical) |
| • Wearing apparel | Actual dollar amount used |
| • Other supplies | Pounds of laundry |
| • Labor | Number of deliveries |
| Mail room | Reclassify to administration |
| Maintenance | Square feet or work orders by cost center |
| Maintenance of facilities | Actual expense to buildings or square feet |
| Materials distribution | Number of deliveries |
| Materials processing | Combine with central sterilization |
| Medical records | Per discharge |
| Nursing administration | Nursing employees |
| Nursing education administration | Reclassify to nursing |
| Pastoral care | Patient days |
| Personnel | Per hour or per number of employees |
| Planning | Combine with administration |
| Plant operations | Square feet by cost center |
| Plant security | Accumulated direct cost |
| Printing | Sample of services rendered to each cost center |
| Purchasing | Number of requisitions |
| Quality assurance/utilization review | Gross revenue |
| Receiving and stores | Number of deliveries |
| Statutory fringe benefits | |
| • Reclassify FICA to a separate cost center | Gross salary |
| • Reclassify remainder to personnel | Per hour or per employee |
| Tumor registry | Reclassify to medical records |
| Volunteers | Time spent |

*Allocation of Indirect and Allocated Costs to Procedures*

Next, allocation data are needed to assign indirect and allocated costs to procedures. Four allocation algorithms are generally available in most cost management software programs to perform this allocation process. These algorithms are:

1. per procedure
2. direct labor time
3. revenue
4. total direct costs

The per-procedure algorithm allocates costs equally to each procedure. For example, if $1,000 is to be allocated and the total procedure volume is 500, each procedure will receive $2 ($1,000 divided by 500) of allocated costs. The major disadvantage of this algorithm is that procedures with low direct costs may absorb a disproportionate share of allocated costs, possibly making them appear expensive and inefficiently produced (for example, a procedure with $.50 of direct costs absorbing $2 of allocated costs).

The direct-labor-time algorithm allocates costs to a procedure based on allocated costs per the amount of direct labor time consumed by the procedure. For example, suppose a particular cost center has $1,000 of costs to allocate and total direct labor minutes of 4,000. For each labor minute, $.25 ($1,000 divided by 4,000) of allocated costs are assigned to a procedure. For a procedure having 30 minutes of direct labor time, $7.50 of allocated costs would be assigned. The algorithm is recommended when direct labor accounts for the majority of procedure costs or when a cost center's indirect costs are mostly labor (for example, manager and supervisor salaries).

The revenue algorithm allocates costs to procedures based on allocated costs per dollar of revenue. For example, suppose a particular cost center has $1,000 to allocate and total revenues of $10,000. For each dollar of revenue, $.10 ($1,000 divided by $10,000) of allocated costs are assigned to a procedure. For a procedure with a unit of revenue of $50, $5 of allocated costs would be assigned.

This algorithm has two disadvantages. First, there is generally only a minimal correlation between revenues and costs. Second, it cannot be used on procedures that are not charged for.

The total-direct-cost algorithm allocates costs to procedures based on allocated costs per dollar of direct cost. For example, suppose a particular cost center has $1,000 to allocate and total direct costs of $20,000.

For each dollar of direct cost, $.05 ($1,000 divided by $20,000) of allocated costs are assigned to a procedure. For a procedure with direct costs of $100, $5 of allocated costs would be assigned. This algorithm is generally the fairest and least controversial way to assign indirect and overhead costs to procedures.

Depending on each specific situation, the appropriate algorithm should be selected for each cost center. The remaining step is to enter each selected algorithm into the cost management computer system. All known systems contain preprogrammed logic routines to perform most, if not all four, of the algorithms.

Once all allocation requirements are satisfied and entered into the system, the allocation routines can be executed, producing the following reports:

- edit reports to verify the existence and accuracy of the data inputs
- procedure resource and cost profile reports, reflecting fully absorbed costs

These reporting outputs should be thoroughly reviewed for reasonableness and completeness. The task force project director is responsible for the initial review. After this review step, the resource and cost information may be accessed by the other applications (for example, case-type costing, flexible budgeting) of the cost management system to test interfaces and other functions.

## REASONABLENESS TESTING

Reasonableness testing measures the validity of the procedure resource and cost standards. A two-step approach is generally recommended, covering:

1. individual procedures
2. the total cost center

### Individual Procedures

To ascertain the reasonableness of the hospital's procedure resource and cost standards, comparisons must be made with available independent standards. Generally, in this process, only total direct labor time is compared, since direct labor usually accounts for a majority of a procedure's costs. When doing comparisons on a procedure-to-procedure basis, geographic location, levels of activity (volumes), differing brands of equipment, and organizational factors generally make the comparisons of indirect labor, labor rates, and supply item usage and cost difficult to do and generally invalid.

The above comparative process is intended to highlight aberrant data. If the aberrations are significant enough (for example, reflecting more than a 25 percent difference), investigative action may be warranted. Significant differences do not mean that the hospital's standards are wrong. However, they may confirm operational inefficiencies previously documented during the cost center operations documentation process or may highlight ones previously not discovered. By following up on operational inefficiencies—for example, by replacing outdated equipment or implementing a new scheduling system—significant reductions in operating costs may be achieved. This adds tangible value to the cost management project, even before it is fully implemented. Multihospital systems may have an advantage in this step, since they are, in reality, developing a self-contained comparative database. By comparing data among their member hospitals' cost centers, they may be able to identify and establish more efficient operational structures.

If there appears to be no rational basis for the differences found in procedure resource usage, the technical estimates may have to be redone, or each procedure may have to be brought into line with industry standards. In either case, significant differences must be brought to the attention of the relevant cost center managers and the task force and their possible impact on the cost management system's outputs and utility. Investigative actions must then be pursued to correct errors and render the system valid.

## Total Cost Center

To ascertain the reasonableness of standards for the cost center, the following categories of information are produced by the cost management system for each cost center:

- variable and fixed labor hours, by skill level and type (for example, productive and nonproductive)
- separate variable and fixed supply and other dollar amounts
- total capital-related dollars

Each of these outputs represents an "earned" amount. That is, based on the control period's volumes and each procedure's standard resource and cost consumption, the cost center should have used specific resources and incurred specific costs to meet that period's level and mix of production.

As a final check on the validity and appropriateness of the standards, cost center control period resources and costs should be compared with and reconciled to earned amounts. Again, to facilitate this process, the following matching data from the control period are required:

- variable and fixed labor hours, by skill level and type (for example, vacation, sick, holiday)
- variable and fixed supply and other dollar amounts
- total capital-related dollars

The control period's fixed and variable resource and cost data were classified and summarized during the initial data-gathering organizational steps. A reconciliation worksheet is now developed to calculate and document the differences between earned and control period amounts. The worksheet should accommodate the lowest level of detail available from the cost management system and the control period's records. This may be as fine as general ledger subaccount detail, or it may be a single gross-dollar amount. Labor hours should, however, be listed by skill level to highlight specific staffing problems. Some software programs may have a built-in reconciliation worksheet capability, thereby obviating the worksheet development process.

All applicable data are entered onto the worksheet or into the cost management system, and variances are calculated for each line item. Significant variances are then investigated to determine their cause and, where necessary, to develop corrective action plans (reduce staffing, replace equipment, etc.).

The significance of a variance depends on two factors: its absolute amount and its percentage in relation to the control period's total amount. For example, $10,000 may seem significant in absolute amount, but it may be insignificant if it represents only six percent of the total control period's costs for the line item. Before any reconciliations take place, a threshold of significance should be defined by the task force project director and approved by the task force. Variance thresholds of greater than $10,000 or 10 percent are commonly used. All thresholds should be consistently applied to avoid claims of unfair treatment and favoritism.

If variances are within threshold guidelines, the quality of the standards is assumed to be high. Standards should not be adjusted to reflect control-period values for performance-monitoring purposes. To do so would invalidate the standards. However, for product-costing purposes, the standards may be adjusted to reflect the costs of actual operational performance. If the variances are outside the threshold guidelines, investigative actions should be initiated to verify the completeness, quality, and integrity of the standards data.

Many times, significant variances arise from such flow and capacity issues as outdated equipment and poor scheduling. These variances can usually be confirmed by reviewing the responses of the operations documentation questionnaire. A plan to correct the relevant flow and capacity issues and produce cost savings should then be formulated.

Often, the exclusion of major activities (for example, assessments or consultations) for which no historical volumes exist may cause a variance. Again, the operations documentation questionnaires should be checked to confirm the presence or absence of these items. In this case, standards for currently costed procedures should not be adjusted; otherwise they will be distorted. New procedures should be added to the cost center to reflect the major activities and to facilitate accurate costing, performance evaluation, and budgeting applications. In the short term—for product costing purposes—the standards may be adjusted to absorb the costs of these activities.

Finally, investigations may lead to the conclusion that a cost center may be basically inefficient or overstaffed. In this case, the cost center manager must be consulted to discuss the situation. If it is agreed that the cost center is overstaffed, a plan to reduce staffing should be developed.

During reasonableness testing, the task force should be kept informed of significant findings and potential cost-reduction opportunities. This will indicate the considerable value of the cost management system, even before it is fully implemented.

All changes resulting from the reasonableness testing process are now documented, quantified, and entered into the software program. Edit reports are produced to verify that all appropriate changes were made. Finally, cost center resource and cost reports are distributed to the cost center managers for their review and acceptance. Except for future enhancements and maintenance, this signals the end of the cost center manager's involvement in the data-gathering process.

## STANDARDS MAINTENANCE

A cost management system's procedure resource and cost standards must be updated periodically to maintain them as an effective management tool. For existing procedures, this entails updating individual procedure resource usage and unit costs. However, as new services are added (for example, a lithotripter), as transaction systems are implemented (for example, a patient classification system), or as additional cost centers develop procedure standards, new procedure resource and cost profile standards must be documented and incorporated into the cost management system database.

Generally, it is recommended that procedure standards be reviewed and updated annually. In periods of high inflation, it is recommended that resource unit costs be updated more frequently (for example, semiannually). The updating process involves a review of existing procedures' standards with the relevant cost center managers.

Significant factors that may change a procedure's production process and cost include:

- new major equipment
- addition or discontinuance of services
- renovations in physical layout
- engagement of a new major materials supplier
- implementation of a scheduling or order-entry results reporting system

If the cost center manager and the individual responsible for the hospital's cost management system agree that existing procedure standards no longer accurately reflect the current production process and costs, the procedure standards may have to be redefined. Large efficiency, rate, or volume/mix variances generally confirm the need to update standards or to correct chronic production problems. Technical-estimate or industrial engineering data-gathering methodologies are recommended to update or develop new procedure standards.

### SUMMARY

Procedure profile resource and cost standards are a vital component of a cost management system. The quality of the standards will have a profound effect on the accuracy and usefulness of the cost management system's applications. Clearly, the quality of such standards must be maintained at a high level if the hospital is to achieve its goals and objectives.

# chapter 8

# Developing Product Resource Consumption Profiles

## INTRODUCTION

This chapter addresses the second major data-collection activity in the implementation phase of a cost management system—the development of product resource consumption profiles. The process of developing these profiles raises several questions. Is there a "standard" product measure? Are DRGs reliable product measures? How does one monitor and control physicians' treatment patterns? How does one use historical treatment data? Is there such a thing as a "standard" treatment pattern? If so, how is it developed? These questions are addressed in this chapter.

Since the implementation of diagnosis related groups (DRGs), clinicians, consumers, and hospital managers have expressed concern over their implications for the practice of medicine. The Medicare Prospective Payment System increased this concern, because it introduced financial risk by using DRGs as the basis for payment. PPS has in fact altered the traditional roles of hospitals and physicians. Previously, the physician served as the advocate of a patient regarding treatment. However, with the advent of PPS, hospitals have had to become increasingly concerned with the financial impact of treating patients, and physicians are now caught in the middle—between the hospital's concern with financial risk and their own traditional role of patient advocate. And the concern about risk-based payment systems is reflected in the new cliches that have developed—cookbook medicine, lines of credit for individual patients, etc.

In actuality, few hospitals have scrutinized physicians' treatment of individual patients to any great extent. Yet PPS—through its outlier provisions—recognizes that certain patients may have special and unusual care needs. In contrast, most hospitals regard DRG payments as reflecting the average cost of care required by patients—by definition, some patients are below average while others are above.

Many hospitals calculate the cost of care for individual patients (hospital products) and then report their cost of care by case type, physician, and payer. Initially, most hospitals determine product costs using ratio of cost-to-charges (RCC); they then move toward more accurate cost measures, such as relative value units (RVUs) or detailed procedural cost standards. Hospital management typically screens products, in total and by payer, for profitability. Profitability by product is a function of several variables—overall hospital costs, efficient treatment of patients, third-party payment terms, etc.

Next, a cursory analysis is conducted to determine why certain products are profitable and others are unprofitable. If overall hospital costs are high—as compared with the budget plan or industry norms—functional cost center managers are pressured to reduce costs, through staffing reductions, lower supplier costs, or fewer capital expenditures. If one payer proves problematic, the hospital may attempt to alter its patient mix—through outreach programs in more favorable geographic areas, by closing emergency rooms and clinics, by aggressively seeking out commercial third-party payer arrangements, etc.

Hospitals perform a similar evaluation of physician costs and profitability, by product and in total. If a physician's overall profitability is poor, the payer mix among the physician's patients is examined to determine its impact on the physician's profitability.

Many hospitals evaluate physician costs, by product and payer, at either the cost-center or the procedure level of detail—depending on the hospital's costing methodology and the capabilities of its cost management system's case mix reporting capabilities. In this process, they are comparing the clinical practice patterns of physicians on theoretically similar (from a clinical and demographic-attribute standpoint) patients.

Most hospital executives have now developed this type of information on at least a rudimentary basis, but they have not actively used it to work with physicians in monitoring or attempting to alter physician practice patterns. There are two reasons for this:

1. General improvements in clinical efficiency—reduced length of stay, fewer tests, etc.—do not necessarily result in increased profitability. With many payers still on a fee-for-service basis—with or without a negotiated percentage discount—reduced volumes translate into reduced incremental revenues. If incremental revenues exceed incremental costs, reduced volumes translate into reduced profitability. Ethically, to maximize profitability, hospitals and physicians cannot improve clinical efficiency for fixed-price patients while maintaining the status quo for clinical excesses for fee-for-service patients. However, as more payers transfer risks to hospitals, through fixed prices or capitated payments, the hesitancy on the part of hospitals to improve clinical efficiency should decrease.

2. Some hospitals view clinical practices in terms of narrowly defined incremental costs. For example, if one physician reduces the number of chest x-rays on all patients within a DRG by one, there would normally be no decrease in staffing, benefits, and depreciation, and there would be only a nominal decrease in film costs. The hospitals view the potential return—reduced incremental costs—as not justifying the implications of attempting to alter an individual physician's clinical practice patterns. However, this view does not justify the abdication of responsibility for monitoring and improving clinical efficiency on a hospitalwide basis. In fact, if products with significant volumes are challenged for medical care standards—a two-view chest x-ray upon admission, a complete complement of lab tests, etc.—noticeable decreases in resource consumption and resultant cost reductions are attainable.

## THE DEFINITION AND SELECTION PROCESS

By virtue of their environment, hospitals are faced with defining product classification-attribute criteria to meet a variety of cost management applications and the needs of a multidiscipline group of users. In this initial section, we focus on the following tasks required to establish these criteria as a basis for developing product resource consumption profiles:

- defining product and product-line classification attributes
- identifying product groupings
- selecting products

## Defining Product and Product-Line Classification Attributes

A full-function cost management system will provide a hospital with the financial and clinical information, by product or product-line, required to achieve its strategic decision making, contracting, and clinical treatment monitoring objectives. Each of these objectives has a different set of product attribute definitions associated with it, and the cost management system must be responsive to those differences.

The selection of product attribute definitions—that is, a product's clinical and demographic characteristics—is generally dependent upon three internal and external environmental needs:

1. need for strategic planning and budgeting applications
2. need to respond to competitive market pressures
3. need to monitor physician resource usage

The unique aspects of defining outpatient products and product lines are examined in a later context.

### Strategic Planning and Budgeting Applications

Strategic planning and budgeting applications generally require the selection of product classification attributes that are meaningful and accurate from an activity-forecasting perspective—relative to product lines, clinical programs, etc.—and that can be used to calculate contractual allowance and cash flow projections—DRGs for Medicare inpatients, obstetric services for an HMO contract, etc.

For example, strategic decisions generally cannot be made at the DRG level because individual DRGs do not represent segments of a hospital's business and are too numerous (almost 500) to forecast accurately on an individual basis. Therefore, the concept of strategic program units (SPUs) has been developed to represent the true lines of the business of a hospital and to provide a manageable number of business units. In some instances, major diagnostic categories (MDCs) may represent SPUs, for example, Cardiology—MDC 05, Diseases and Disorders of the Circulatory System. In other instances, several MDCs may combine into an SPU, for example, OB/GYN services—MDC 13, Disease and Disorders of the Female Reproductive System; MDC 14, Pregnancy, Childbirth and the Puerperium; and MDC 15, Newborns and other Neonates. Other SPUs, such as those for pediatrics or oncology, are combinations of individual DRGs across MDCs. Finally, SPUs may be an aggregation of subsets of DRGs, such as the trauma SPU defined by admission type, regardless of DRG. A cost management system must be able to define resource consumption (and costs) by SPUs to enable the hospital to evaluate its products for investment, marketing, and physician recruitment purposes.

### Responses to Competitive Market Pressures

The response to competitive market pressures begins by selecting the product classification attributes required to react to a direct solicitation for contracted services—for example, an HMO bid based on a per-discharge payment by DRG—or to market services, such as obstetric services to a specific geographic area, proactively. Since no single product measure is universally appropriate for all insurers or for the health care industry as a whole, hospitals may need to address any number of market-defined or internally defined product measures.

Currently, most product pricing decisions are made on the basis of DRG product definitions. Medicare has adopted DRGs as the basis of payment, using historical requirements for Medicare patient resource consumption. Many other third-party payers have also adopted DRGs as the basis for product definition and for payment, since hospitals are already using them for product definition. Other payers use other product definitions as the basis of payment—a flat rate per diem, regardless of illness; medical-versus-surgical patients, paid on a per-diem or per-discharge basis; or a series of payer-defined SPUs, such as OB/GYN services, pediatrics, etc., paid on a per-diem or per-discharge basis. The ability to establish alternative product definitions depends on the type of clinical and demographic data captured by the hospital for each patient.

### Monitoring of Physician Resource Usage

The process of evaluating clinical practices must be supported by the cost management system. The monitoring of physician resource usage requires the selection of product classification attributes that define products in both a clinically meaningful and a consistent manner. In addition, a severity-of-illness measure, to enhance product classification schemes, is desirable. By structuring attribute definitions in this way, analyses of physician treatment protocols can be based on valid, acceptable classification schemes.

DRGs were initially designed to account for length-of-stay variations among patients. However, clinicians have challenged the ability of DRGs to provide a truly homogeneous patient group on the basis of length of stay or total resource requirements. They are concerned that DRGs do not accurately measure a patient's illness level, thus making patients within a DRG clinically incomparable. Numerous patient classification schemes are available to enhance or replace the DRG methodology for clinical monitoring purposes. Among the more widely known classification schemes are:

- Disease Staging
- Medical Index Severity Grouping System
- Severity of Illness Index
- Patient Management Categories

In the following paragraphs, we present an overview of these four classification methods. More detailed information on their composition and applicability can be found in *Health Care Financing Review* (1984 Annual Supplement, Health Care Financing Administration, Baltimore, Maryland).

*Disease Staging*

Disease Staging, developed by Joseph S. Gonnella, M.D., dean of Thomas Jefferson Medical College, together with SysteMetrics, Inc., uses patient clinical data in the medical record after discharge to assign patients to one of approximately 400 disease categories (pneumonia, diabetes, etc.). It also uses these data to assess the biological progression (stage) of the disease (generally), ranging from Stage I, disease with no complications or minimal severity, to Stage IV, death caused by the disease. This mechanism provides approximately 1,600 patient groupings of clinically similar patients.

Disease Staging may be used as an alternative to DRGs for clinical evaluation, or it may enhance DRGs as a measure of severity. Its strongest attributes are its objectivity, its use of readily available data, and its simple and low-cost implementation. Its drawbacks relate to its method for determining disease specificity (all Stage I patients are not alike; they vary by disease category) and its conceptual development method (using theoretical definitions of severity levels, not statistical evaluations of historical resource consumption trends).

## Medical Index Severity Grouping System

The Medical Index Severity Grouping System (MEDISGROUPS), developed by MediQual, uses an evaluation system to measure patient severity concurrent with admission and hospitalization. The system tallies assigned weights for key clinical findings—such as tissue swelling or intercranial bleeding as noted in a radiological exam—to establish a severity score, ranging from Severity Group 0, no key findings, to Severity Group 5, critical findings with organ failure. The major advantage of MEDISGROUPS is its accurate and straightforward applicability to DRGs—each DRG can be stratified from 0 to 5 without regard to disease. Its major drawback is its implementation cost; it requires human intervention to identify key clinical findings within a patient chart and to enter this data into the MEDISGROUPS system software.

## Severity of Illness Index

The Severity of Illness Index, developed by Susan Horn, is comparable with MEDISGROUPS because it rates a patient's severity based on a tallied score. The index evaluates patients using a score of one to four for each of seven criteria—stage of the disease, complications, interacting conditions, dependency on hospital staff, nonoperating-room-like support systems, rate of recovery, and remaining impairment. The composite average score, ranging from one to four, is the Severity of Illness Index. Clinical studies have shown that the index is a reliable measure of resource consumption and, therefore, a highly useful tool in stratifying products. The drawback of the index is in its operation—it is somewhat subjective and requires significant human intervention, by specifically trained "raters," on a concurrent basis.

## Patient Management Categories

Finally, Patient Management Categories, developed by Wanda Young at Blue Cross of Western Pennsylvania, attempts to categorize patients based on their clinical diagnostic and treatment paths. The category groupings begin with the symptoms manifested upon admission and progress through the process of diagnosis, treatment, and outcome, in contrast to DRGs that retrospectively look at discharge clinical data. This system comes closest to prescribing a clinical protocol to classify patients and thus can serve as an alternative to DRGs. As the system is not yet fully implemented, however it is difficult to assess its strengths and weaknesses.

### Identifying Product Groupings

When implementing a comprehensive cost management system, it is critical to address product and product-line measures. To do this, the hospital must identify the users of product information, identify the products and product lines to be defined, and develop the appropriate classification methodology. Based on current experience, most hospitals are using some form of SPU along with DRGs. Several large institutions now analyze patient data using stratified DRGs, Disease Staging, MEDISGROUPS, or the Severity of Illness Index.

An overriding consideration in defining products for clinical analysis purposes is the volume of data being analyzed. While any severity measure applied to DRGs increases the homogeneity of the groupings, it greatly reduces the number of patients in a given cell (for example, DRG by severity). Therefore, because there are fewer occurrences in each cell, historical norms may lose their statistical validity. In practical application, a large percentage of all discharges will occur in fewer than 50 case types. Therefore, generally, any severity stratification should be applied only to these 50 case types.

Another critical issue in defining products and product lines is in the determination of the appropriate manner to address outpatients. Because PPS and DRGs relate only to inpatients, hospitals have been slow to include outpatients in their product analyses. Moreover, in most hospitals, the volume of outpatient records to be processed is excessive when compared with the dollar volume of outpatient services. When considering the inclusion of outpatient products in a cost management system, two factors must be evaluated.

1. outpatient product definition
2. relationship, if any, to inpatient stays

Separate outpatient products may be designed in a number of ways, including:

- clinical service
- diagnostic clusters
- ambulatory patient groups (APGs)

Defining outpatients by clinical service would occur at the point of registration and treatment by indicating to which SPU an outpatient's visit relates. For example, outpatient registration would assign a mammography to the SPU, Women's and Children's Health, or to a similar SPU. This method requires that outpatient registration personnel understand and be able to ascertain a given patient's SPU grouping. Normally, a series of SPU code-grouping guidelines is established to provide consistency and accuracy in the process.

Diagnostic clusters (DCs) represent a retrospective grouping method. The DCs are 104 predefined groupings based on the International Classification of Diseases—Ninth Revision—Clinical Modification (ICD-9-CM) codes. Examples of these groupings are General Medical Examination, Acute Upper Respiratory Infection, and Prenatal and Postnatal Care. The DC grouping logic is completely analagous to that of the DRG "Grouper." Therefore, DCs may be linked with associated inpatient SPUs to combine both inpatient and outpatient products.

A variation of the DC grouping methodology is the use of ambulatory patient groups (APGs). In this method, patients are assigned to APGs, using a decision tree that includes ICD-9-CM codes and background information (initial visit, referral information, etc.). There are 154 APGs aggregated into 14 major ambulatory categories (MACs).

Each of the above methods can assign a unique episode of outpatient care to a specific product or product line. If this is sufficient for the hospital's purposes, it will be easy to integrate outpatients into its cost management system.

As more third parties seek to transfer risk to hospitals, they are moving away from paying separately for each episode of care—an admission, a preadmission diagnostic visit, a home-health agency visit, etc.—and toward the use of bundled services—either by spell of illness or by capitation. In these instances, it is appropriate for a hospital to define a product that combines inpatient and outpatient services. The only way to accomplish this is to have on financial and medical records patient identification (number) schemes that are unique to either a patient spell of illness or a patient (beneficiary). To do this, hospitals must assess the payment terms of major third-party payers and align their patient identification (number) schemes with those payment terms, that is, using unique patient numbers for each episode of care, spell of illness, or enrolled beneficiary.

Regardless of which application—strategic planning and budgeting, responding to market pressures, or monitoring physicians—the hospital wishes to pursue, its cost management system must be able to accept any combination of product classification attributes.

## Selecting Products

After product and product-line attributes have been defined and patient groupings have been identified, the process of selecting products for profiling begins. Paring down the number of products or product lines is generally necessary to minimize computer hardware capacity constraints, standards development and maintenance efforts, and software processing time.

To facilitate the process, the hospital's cost management system will be required to produce historical product or product-line listings that include information on

- volume
- total gross revenues and costs
- net revenues, variable costs, and profitability

This information would then be reviewed by the end users of the product—planners, financial personnel, or physicians—to determine which individual products or product lines have significant activity, revenue, or cost to justify the development of resource consumption profiles. For physician monitoring applications, 80/20 selection rules generally do not apply. The supporting rationale is that activity below the top 10 to 25 products is too infrequent—generally less than 50 cases per year at 300- to 500-bed hospitals—to be clinically meaningful from a treatment perspective.

For products or product lines not selected for individual standards development, new classification attribute criteria must be developed to collapse them into generic groupings—such as MDCs for strategic planning or budgeting applications—or to exclude them entirely for standards development (for example, in the case of low-volume products for physician treatment monitoring applications).

## PRODUCT RESOURCE CONSUMPTION PROFILE STANDARDS

### Data Sources

After the product selection process is completed, the resource consumption profile development process begins. As noted previously, the basis of the product resource consumption profiles is the historical treatment patterns experienced at the hospital. In some circumstances, the relevant historical proprietary information may be supplemented by regional or national product resource consumption databases. For example, if the hospital is planning to introduce a new clinical service, it obviously would have no history on which to base the types and amount of resources to be consumed by that classification of patient. However, by accessing a regional or national database, the requisite resource consumption profiles, based on hospitals serving populations with similar demographic characteristics, such as age, sex, and socio-economic factors, and closely approximating the hospital's expected experience, can be formulated. Other circumstances in which a regional or national database may be used include those when physicians desire input from neutral sources to develop standard treatment protocols or when a hospital wants to alter practice patterns based on practice norms accepted outside its particular institutional philosophy.

## Types of Applications

Next, using the hospital's cost management system, a resource consumption profile—detailing the types and amount of services consumed by each individual procedure—is produced for each product. At this point, the resource consumption profile development process becomes a dual approach, based on two types of applications:

1. marketing, planning, and budgeting applications
2. physician resource monitoring applications

### Marketing, Planning, and Budgeting

Marketing, planning, and budgeting applications generally recognize product profiles in terms of average historical resource consumption—regardless of strides toward optimal treatment efficiency. The rationale supporting the use of historical averages for these applications is three-fold:

1. Hospitals treat a wide variety of patients, including those that require significantly more or fewer resources (outliers) than other patients. By recognizing the historical fact that the hospital will treat patients who will consume more or fewer resources than average, management can make better forecasts of expected procedure volumes, cost center requirements, and profitability.
2. The hospital's physicians do not provide identical treatment regimens. Therefore, perceived efficiencies in treatment—from high-ad-

mitting specialized physicians—may be offset by other physicians from other, related specialties who admit and treat similar types of patients.

3. The marketing, pricing, and budgeting applications must reflect what will happen, not what the hospital would like to see happen, in order to have utility for their end users.

Thus, the historical average resource consumption profiles generated by the hospital's case mix reporting system become the resource consumption profile standards for budgeting, planning, and marketing applications. No paring down on the number of procedures (for example, an 80/20 analysis) within each product or product line is necessary, since all procedures are required to cost accurately a product or product line and to forecast all procedure volumes for the cost center.

Breakdowns of products by payer within a product line—for contractual allowance and cash flow projection purposes—is generally accomplished by applying historical payer mix percentages, supplemented by contractual information (for example, from a newly obtained HMO contract).

## Physician Resource Monitoring

Physician resource monitoring applications require resource consumption profiles that reflect desired treatment patterns and are typically less detailed as to the number of procedures. Additionally, to be developed, they require an in-depth involvement on the part of physicians and clinicians. Product-line managers and nurse clinicians should also be involved.

The most efficient way to create this involvement is to form a committee that will take responsibility for the development of profiles. Each historical average resource consumption profile report, listing the types and amounts of procedures consumed is then reviewed by the committee. Each procedure is challenged as to its appropriateness and amount of usage in a treatment regimen for each product being reviewed. In this process, a derivation of average resource consumption profile reports may be employed. This derivation shows average resource consumption by procedure and by each day of stay—a CBC on the first day of stay, IV therapy on the second day, physical therapy on the eighth day, and so on. This day-by-day information enables the committee to analyze the treatment process and to highlight the progression of treatment, not just the result. Once a treatment profile (protocol) for a particular product has been agreed upon, it can be entered into the cost management system to facilitate treatment variance reporting.

Due to the sensitivity of establishing treatment profiles and the fact that each patient has some unique characteristics, regardless of the number and type of classification attributes, many hospitals choose to involve physicians gradually in the review of treatment variances. At first, treatment variance reports are provided to physicians for informational purposes only. Then, by utilizing the committees previously formed to develop the profiles, forums are made available to monitor and maintain the profiles and to police those physicians with consistently atypical treatment patterns that cannot be explained.

## SUMMARY

To be effective, a cost management system must recognize the hospital's unique definition of products and product lines and support multiple definitions for multiple management purposes. It is not sufficient, in most instances, to allow the hospital simply to define resource consumption by DRG alone. Many hospitals will need a cost management system that provides multiple product definitions for each patient— each with standard resource consumption profiles—that may be aggregated in several ways to support strategic, clinical, and pricing decisions.

Product definition and standard (protocol) setting for resource consumption profiles are areas of increasing interest to hospitals and physicians. Applications of this chapter's information and guidelines will clearly be subject to significant changes as the industry progresses further toward product-line management and better research and development in product-line classification systems.

# part III

# APPLICATIONS OF COST MANAGEMENT INFORMATION

# *Organizational Structures to Achieve Cost Management*

## INTRODUCTION

In the previous chapters, we addressed the value and benefits of cost management, how cost management systems are designed and implemented, and how hospitals can improve their competitive position by using cost management information. As noted earlier, a cost management system is not an isolated, stand-alone system that can be simply "dropped" into a hospital. Of the many factors that have to be considered, the hospital's organizational structure is of particular importance.

To accommodate the changes brought about by a cost management philosophy, the hospital's current organizational structure may have to be modified. The result should be an organizational structure that is fully responsive to the needs of the hospital's patients, medical staff, and management, leading to a more cost-effective delivery of care.

In anticipation of a need to refine their current structure, some hospitals address the organizational issue before implementing the cost management system. In these cases, the existing organizational structure is considered to be a constraining factor in the successful implementation of a cost management philosophy. However, most hospitals prefer a more cautious approach to change. In these cases, the potential changes that are foreseen in the current organizational structure are effected during and after the design and implementation of the cost management system.

In any event, regardless of when the organizational issue is addressed, it is vital that top management and the board evaluate and understand the organizational structure issues of cost management. Typically, the following questions are asked in the process of understanding and evaluating a health care organization's delivery structure:

- Who is accountable for developing business plans?
- Who is responsible for marketing and advertising products and services?
- Should we decentralize advertising decisions, or should we centralize them, promoting a common image of the organization?
- What prices do we bid for specific services, individually and packaged?
- What are the physicians' management responsibilities?
- How do we monitor and control clinical treatment regimens within product types?
- For what variances do we hold functional departmental managers responsible?
- What incentives, in terms of compensation and other benefits, do we provide to management for their performance?

The answers to these kinds of questions are critical in the assessment of the organizational structure as a basis for promoting an efficient and effective cost management environment.

The organizational structures that currently can be found in hospitals include functional, product-line, and matrix structures. In this chapter, we present and analyze the key issues to be addressed when determining the appropriate organizational structure needed to complement a cost management philosophy and to achieve its objectives.

## KEY ORGANIZATIONAL ISSUES

Before examining the various organizational structures available to the health care industry, several key organizational issues should be addressed. First, management must understand the definition and purpose of an organizational structure. This includes identifying its objectives and ascertaining to what degree the hospital's existing structure meets its current and future needs. If the hospital decides a change in its organizational structure is necessary, currently available structures— functional management structure, product-line structure, and matrix structure—and the environments in which they operate most effectively should be reviewed. Then, if appropriate, a new structure may be established.

The existing structures of hospitals and other health care organizations are generally reflected in their organizational charts and their policy and procedure manuals. The organizational chart represents a series of activities and processes comprising four key components (Child 1977, 10):

1. description of the allocation of tasks and responsibilities to individuals and departments throughout the organization
2. designation of formal reporting relationships, including the number of levels in the hierarchy and the span of control of managers and supervisors
3. identification of the grouping of individuals in departments and the grouping of departments in the total organization
4. the design of various systems to ensure effective communication, coordination, and integration of effort in both vertical and horizontal directions

Many factors determine how an organization should structure itself to deliver its products and services. However, the major factor is recognition of a dominant competitive issue.

A dominant competitive issue represents what the organization has to do to satisfy its customers, to stay ahead of competitors, and to earn economic profits. Top managers interpret the dominant competitive issue in their industry and derive goals from it. In an industry such as the manufacture of electronic calculators, the dominant competitive issue is new product innovation. In the trucking industry, the dominant competitive issue is timely and reliable service. Customers choose a trucking firm based on its ability to provide service when needed. Organizational goals will thus reflect the desire to provide this service to customers. The dominant competitive issue and goals depend on the environment of the firm, and may include such things as low prices, product efficiency, innovation, marketing, product quality, or a combination of several factors. (Daft 1986, 213)

In the health care industry, the dominant competitive issue may vary by area of the country, locale (urban versus rural), and other factors. However, the dominant competitive issue in most areas is perceived to be "market share." To increase or maintain market share, hospitals must be cost-competitive, manage their delivery mechanisms effectively, and deliver high-quality services. However, many hospitals have not followed this approach. Since the inception of the Medicare Prospective Payment System, many hospitals have blindly set forth to maintain or increase their market share, regardless of their cost position or the relative quality of their services. However, now most of these hospitals are reconsidering this approach, as the buyers of health care become more sophisticated and are asking for more competitive prices and differentiation of quality. To respond to these demands, hospitals need to adopt a cost management philosophy. And to make implementation of that philosophy a success, alternative organizational structures may need to be reviewed to determine the one that can most effectively leverage the information the cost management system provides to protect and expand market share.

## TYPES OF ORGANIZATIONAL STRUCTURES

### Functional

Traditional organizational structures in the health care field are generally based on functional skills. Nurses report to the nursing director, laboratory technicians to the laboratory director, and so on. Over the years, this organizational structure has served hospitals well. It has been responsive to the growth of technical staff, has served the clinical gatekeepers, and has provided good vertical linkages between policies and procedures. In general, the functional structure groups people, technical functions, and activities together with their control functions.

The functional form of organization is best when the dominant competitive issue and goals of the organization stress functional expertise, efficiency, and quality. Employees in each department adopt similar values, goals, and orientations. Similarity encourages collaboration, efficiency, and quality within the function, but makes coordination and cooperation with other departments more difficult. The functional structure places the emphasis on expertise within functions rather than on horizontal coordination. Even with task forces and integrators, the primary allegiance of employees will be toward the goals of their own departments rather than toward cooperation with other departments. . . .

. . . The functional structure is most effective in a relatively stable environment. Vertical mechanisms provide coordination and integration. Within the organization, employees are committed to achieving the goals of their respective functional departments. Planning and budgeting is by function and reflects the cost of resources used in each department. Promotion up the hierarchy is normally on the basis of experience and expertise within the function (e.g., marketing, engineering). The information and linkage processes are mostly vertical and include the hierarchy, rules, and planning.

One strength of the functional structure is that it promotes economy of scale within functions. Economy of scale means that all employees are located in the same place and can share facilities. Producing all products in a single plant, for example, enables the plant to acquire the latest machinery. Constructing only one facility instead of a separate facility for each product line reduces duplication and waste. The functional structure also promotes in-depth skill development of employees. Employees are exposed to a range of functional activities within their own department. The functional form of structure is best for small to medium-sized organizations when there is only one or a few products produced. (Daft 1986, 226–228)

The organizational characteristics associated with a functional structure are summarized in Table 9–1.

**Product-Line**

As an alternative to the functional structure, a growing number of hospitals are adopting a product-line organizational structure borrowed

**Table 9–1** Summary of Functional Organization Characteristics for Health Care Organizations

Health care environment:
  Environmental considerations: Low to moderate uncertainty and minimal competition
  Dominant competitive issue: Technical specialization and cost efficiency

Management systems:
  Planning, budgeting, and control: General ledger basis—budget, statistical reports, and unit cost control
  Influence: Department managers
  Promotion: On basis of functional expertise
  Information flow: Vertical (hierarchical) flow, top-down technical control, and general management policies and procedures

Strengths
  1. Best in stable environment
  2. Maximizes economies of scale
  3. Supports in-depth skill development
  4. Colleagueship for technical specialists
  5. Best in small to medium-size health care organizations
  6. Best when only limited number of product lines are offered

Weaknesses
  1. Slow response time to environmental changes
  2. Bottlenecks across departmental entities
  3. More difficult interdepartmental coordination
  4. Less innovation
  5. Restricted view of strategic direction
  6. Product priority conflicts

Source: Adapted, by permission of the publisher, from "What Is the Right Organization Structure? Decision Tree Analysis Provides the Answer," by R. Duncan, *Organizational Dynamics*, Winter 1979, p. 64, © 1979 American Management Association, New York. All rights reserved.

---

from their manufacturing counterparts. The term *product-line structure* is used as a generic term for clinical lines of business or service that are self-contained units. (Some health care executives do not like to use the term *product-line* for health care because of its association with assembly-line manufacturing products. Here, we use product line as a generic term to simplify our terminology for discussion purposes. Each institution will, of course adopt the terminology most appropriate in their environments.)

Product lines can be organized by clinical services, diagnosis related groups (DRGs) or groups of DRGs, markets, customers, or major programs. Whereas the functional structure is organized by inputs (resources), the product-line structure is organized by outputs.

> The product form of structure is excellent when the dominant competitive issue and goals of the organization emphasize coordinated action to innovate, satisfy clients, or to maintain a market segment. Environmental uncertainty is moderate to high. Since the self-contained units are often quite small, employees identify with the product line rather than with their own function. Budgeting and planning is on a profit basis, because each product line can be run as a separate business with both costs and income calculated. Managers with influence are those who lead the product division. Promotion into higher management is typically on the basis of management and integration skills rather than on functional expertise. Managers must be able to achieve coordination across functions rather than to be an expert in any single function. The product structure stresses horizontal as well as vertical coordination.
>
> The product structure has several strengths. It is suited to fast change in an unstable environment and provides high product visibility. Since each product is a separate division, clients are able to contact the right division and achieve satisfaction. Coordination across functions is excellent. Each product can adapt to requirements of individual customers or regions. The product structure typically works best in large organizations that have multiple products or services and enough personnel to staff separate functional units.
>
> One disadvantage is the organization loses economies of scale. Instead of 50 research engineers sharing a common facility in a functional structure, 10 engineers may be assigned to each of five product divisions. The critical mass required for in-depth research is lost and physical facilities have to be duplicated for each product line. Another problem is product lines become separate from each other and coordination across product lines can be difficult. In-depth competence and technical specialization are lost in this structure. Employees identify with the product line rather than with a functional specialty. R&D personnel, for example, tend to do applied research to benefit the product line rather than basic research to benefit the entire organization. (Daft 1986, 230–231)

A summary of the characteristics of a product-line organizational structure is presented in Table 9–2.

The issue of whether organizational entities should be grouped by function or by product poses a major dilemma for many health care organizations. Even in other industries, there is still no consensus as to which approach works best in which environment. However, more than 75 percent of all larger organizational entities are structured as product-line organizations.

### Matrix

In a health care organization, the benefits of both functional and product-line structures may be needed. The result is a matrix organiza-

---

**Table 9–2** Summary of Product Organization Characteristics for Health Care Organizations

Health care environment:
  Environmental considerations: Moderate to high uncertainty; competitive
  Dominant competitive issue: Market share (distribution channels and product quality)

Management systems:
  Planning, budgeting, and control: Product-line profit and loss statements
  Influence: Product-line managers
  Promotion: On basis of management skills and profit/loss results
  Information flow: Lateral as well as vertical

Strengths:
  1. Suited to rapidly changing and unstable environments
  2. Client satisfaction—patient is focus for most activities
  3. Easy-to-cross functional lines
  4. Best in large organizations
  5. Best for comprehensive product offerings
  6. Enhanced product image—result of product visibility

Weaknesses:
  1. Loss of economies of scale in departments
  2. More difficult functional coordination across product lines
  3. Deterioration of in-depth competence and technical specialization
  4. Integration and standardization across product lines is difficult
  5. Growth is product oriented—limits new product innovation

*Source:* Adapted, by permission of the publisher, from "What Is the Right Organization Structure? Decision Tree Analysis Provides the Answer," by R. Duncan, *Organizational Dynamics,* Winter 1979, p. 66, © 1979 American Management Association, New York. All rights reserved.

tion. A summary of the characteristics of a matrix organization is presented in Table 9–3.

While the matrix organization solves the product-versus-function dilemma, it has some severe limitations. The most significant limitation is that it results in duplicate reporting responsibilities, that is, on both a horizontal (product) line and a vertical (functional) line.

## Comparative Characteristics

The differences between functional, product-line, and matrix organizations are significant. Health care organizations need to address these differences, given their current environments and specific objectives. Example organizational structure recommendations, based on various criteria, are presented in Table 9–4.

---

**Table 9–3** Summary of Matrix Organization Characteristics for Health Care Organizations

Health care environment:
  Environmental considerations: High uncertainty; highly competitive
  Dominant competitive issue: Dual-market share, technical specialization, and cost efficiency

Management systems:
  Planning, budgeting, and control: Dual systems—by department and product line
  Influence: Joint between department heads and product-line managers
  Promotion: On basis of functional expertise within departments or management/P&L skills across product lines
  Information flow: Direct contact among matrix managers

Strengths:
  1. Addresses coordination necessary to meet demands of changing environment
  2. Flexible use of human resources across product lines
  3. Provides opportunity for functional and marketing skill development
  4. Best in medium-size community hospitals

Weaknesses:
  1. Participants experience dual authority, often causing frustration and confusion
  2. Managers need excellent interpersonal skills and ongoing management training
  3. Managers must understand organization structure and adopt teamwork attitude
  4. Can be time-consuming, with frequent meetings

*Source:* Adapted, by permission of the publisher, from "What Is the Right Organization Structure? Decision Tree Analysis Provides the Answer," by R. Duncan, *Organizational Dynamics,* Winter 1979, p. 71, © 1979 American Management Association, New York. All rights reserved.

**Table 9–4** Example Organizational Structures for Health Care Institutions

| Organization and Environment | Recommended Structure | Responsibilities and Authorities |
|---|---|---|
| General Hospital Rural hospital, 80 beds, sole-community provider, nonprofit organization | Functional structure | Department managers have functional cost control. CEO has pricing and marketing responsibilities. |
| Eastern Medical Center Teaching hospital, tertiary care, 1,200 beds, significant competition, several managed care options, physician-dominated | Product-line structure | Product-line managers are physicians, set up along clinical service lines, with responsibility for pricing, marketing, and cost control. |
| Community Memorial Hospital Comprehensive, community hospital, 350 beds, CEO and COO strongly managed, competitive environment | Matrix structure | Product-line managers are typically young and aggressive, with MBAs, and have marketing responsibilities. Functional managers pursue technical advancement. |

## PRODUCT LINE MANAGEMENT APPLICATIONS

Due to its widespread applicability, the product-line management organizational structure is increasing in popularity among hospitals. There are two primary driving forces behind this trend. The first is the increased emphasis on pricing and marketing. The second, together with the first, is the growing need to control costs. Pricing and marketing requires relatively simple applications of product-line management, compared with that for controlling costs. This is because the collection and manipulation of cost and market data for pricing and marketing requires only limited involvement with employees outside the finance and marketing functions. Thus, we find that many hospitals have developed or are developing cost data for pricing and marketing applications as their initial cost management objective, with the view to extending the effort later to cost control applications. Controlling cost is the larger undertaking because it clearly goes beyond the realm of the finance and marketing functions and requires the participation and commitment of the entire hospital.

Product-line management requires the hospital to:

- identify those who are best able to control the various operational aspects of the hospital—aspects that impact not only expenses but also revenues and net revenues
- clearly delineate responsibility and authority for the components of the cost equation (for example, unit cost and volume)
- hold people accountable for what they have been given the authority and responsibility to control
- monitor the performance of each individual in meeting performance targets

Clearly these objectives require the support of all management levels.

A question top management must address when implementing a product-line management philosophy concerns the relationship of product-line management to its cost management goals and objectives. The following six items represent some of the issues involved:

1. "Cost accounting" for cost control is an effort that requires the participation of the entire hospital. Cost management systems by themselves do not control costs; they merely support management in its efforts to be effective and efficient.
2. A cost management system needs to support the hierarchy and delineation of responsibility in a hospital. It must help managers monitor their performance in their continual effort to manage their responsibilities.
3. A cost management system cannot be implemented solely by the hospital's finance department. The best results are achieved when all disciplines and levels of management participate in the development of the system. For example, having the CEO serve on the cost management task force shows commitment to the success of implementing the system. In our own experience, we have found that those projects that stay on schedule and obtain results have a high degree of commitment from top management. Clearly, management needs to be supportive of a project of this magnitude if it is to be successful.
4. Implementation of a cost management system can be a two- to three-year effort. Many hospitals invest considerable time, energy, and resources in these projects, and they expect large returns as the systems become fully operational and utilized. They should also understand that, depending on the nature of the

project and its priorities, the costs of the system can be reduced significantly during implementation, for example, by adjusting staff levels.

5. Implementing a cost management system is a multifaceted undertaking. There are a variety of starting points, typically in the area or areas of most concern to the hospital. Possible starting points include:

- cost determination to be used for pricing and marketing applications
- reorganization of management (for example, product-line management) to market and manage the hospital's products more effectively, leading to a clearer delineation of responsibility, authority, and accountability, and ultimately to management effectiveness
- cost reduction programs to address immediate cost-competitive problems being experienced in the marketplace and as reflected on the hospital's income statement

6. Cost management is not just a "systems" issue. The purchase and installation of a cost management system and the issuing of reports will not by themselves reduce or manage costs more effectively. In addition, an implementation process is needed that reflects how the hospital is altering its current management philosophy. In short, the hospital's management philosophy is ultimately supported by the cost management system.

A common theme among the above items is that the implementation of a cost management system is a significant undertaking that requires the commitment and support of the board, the hospital's physicians, and top management. A second common theme is the significant overlap between a product-line management organization structure and the cost management system that supports it.

## Organizational Issues

### Defining Product Lines[1]

The first question to be addressed when organizing along product lines is: What are the product lines? Hospitals have taken different

[1]The material in the following discussion of organizational issues has been adapted from "Product-Line Management: Systems and Strategies" by J.G. Nackel and I.W. Kues, *Hospital and Health Services Administration*, pp. 111–114, with permission of American College of Health Care Executives, © March/April 1986.

approaches to defining their products, based on hospital size, specialization, and teaching issues. No single product-line definition is right for every hospital. Product lines can be defined as medical specialty lines, aggregations of DRGs, or other clinical elements specific to the hospital. In any case, however, each product line should be a separate and distinct "business unit" within the hospital. In combination, the business units should be appropriate for the planning, budgeting, monitoring, and controlling of services and for the advertising and marketing of these services to the general public. Each of the business units should be oriented as a profit/loss center.

When establishing the hospital's business units, a key organizational issue concerns the separation of responsibilities according to who controls the various aspects of each product—marketing, cost, delivery, quality, and so on. This issue is especially relevant for services that cross business-unit lines. For example, ancillary services, which most of the business units require, should have a separate responsibility reporting line. Control of these services can be managed through the ancillary service's control of unit cost and the business unit's control of volume usage.

This approach contrasts sharply with that of traditional cost control in hospitals. Many hospital department managers have come to believe that their power and prestige are based on the number of employees and assets they control. This was particularly true under a cost reimbursement system that rewarded hospitals for actual costs incurred rather than for a fixed price per unit of service.

An organization with a cost management emphasis requires a different attitude toward the responsibility function. In a cost management organizational structure, management at all levels (top management, middle managers, supervisors, and staff) must understand that power and prestige are related to performance and that performance is measured in terms of quality service, profitability, efficiency, and effectiveness.

## Identifying Appropriate Managers

The next question is: Who should manage the business units or product lines? The answer will vary by the type of business, teaching and nonteaching responsibilities involved, and by the individual people skills in the organization. For example, teaching hospitals would probably assign physicians as the product-line (business-unit) managers (Table 9–5 lists the pros and cons of physicians as product managers). Community hospitals would be more likely to assign younger, business

**Table 9–5** Physicians as Product Managers

Pros _____

- Physicians are in the best position to directly understand and address the needs of the health care consumer.
- Physicians have power in the organization and the final word in the delivery of all medical care.
- Physicians might provide a more positive image to patients who may find greater comfort or trust in knowing that physicians are managing all components of their care.

Cons _____

- Physicians traditionally have had less influence, skill, or formal authority over nonclinical areas, including finance, housekeeping, billing, and food services.
- Hospital staff may perceive that physicians already have too much power in the hospital, and positioning physicians as product managers may increase this perception or fear.
- Physicians do not tend to be strategically oriented, which product management demands.

*Source:* Reprinted by permission from *Hospitals*, Vol. 60, No. 14, July 20, 1986. Copyright 1986, American Hospital Publishing, Inc.

_____

school graduates with the marketing skills and enthusiasm needed to promote a product line.

Each business-unit manager should report directly to the chief executive officer (CEO) or the chief operating officer (COO). This is important to maintain the continuity of services and the clinical direction of the business, as well as to maintain the autonomy of each individual business unit. If a business unit does not report to the CEO or COO, it should be folded into a different business-unit rather than report to another separate business unit. A business unit manager may decide to delineate additional clinical, operational, or financial responsibilities within the business unit to increase control and accountability.

Once the business units are defined, the business manager should have both the authority and responsibility for the internal profit/loss of the product line. This facilitates the maximization of operating effectiveness within the business unit. Business units managed by operations personnel (rather than physicians) should offer their personnel career advancements to larger or more complex business units. In fact, this kind of transportability across business units should be considered a necessary part of the organizational structure. It allows business managers to learn the different operating units of the hospital and provides a business manager with appropriate training for future career growth. For physician product managers, this may be less appropriate, given their clinical specialty training and their contribution to the organization as a whole.

## Defining Roles and Responsibilities

Product-line manager responsibilities include planning for services (for example, developing a formal business plan), budgeting, and maintaining management control within the business unit. The business plan should be reviewed at the hospital's clinical, operational, and financial levels. When specific marketing actions are identified in the plan, consideration should be given to HMO, PPO, and other managed care activities. The budget should be developed under the product-line manager's responsibility and controlled at the product-line manager level.

This cycle of planning, marketing, budgeting, and control should be consistent across all product lines. The planning process must allow individual business plans to identify the interactive effects between one business line and another, so that changes in technology, clinical practice, and pricing can be assessed across all business units in the organization.

In establishing the product-line management organization, top management must be concerned about practical reporting relationships. In this context, what works in a teaching hospital may not work equally well in a community hospital. In this regard, hospital management should consider the following issues when implementing a product-line management structure:

- The principal product lines should be based on the clinical delivery structure of the organization.
- The span of control at each level of the organization should cover no more than eight to ten functions.
- Staff services, such as information systems, should reflect corporate objectives rather than product-line objectives.
- Staff activities (for example, finance and personnel) should work closely with the departments, but answer to the chief executive officer.

When changing to or supplementing an organizational structure with product-line managers, there may be some managerial conflict. In such situations, it should be remembered that the product-line manager responds to market changes, addresses product needs, and is concerned with coordination and communication across departments, while the functional manager responds to workloads, addresses the need of the particular department, and is concerned with coordination and communication within the department across product lines. An example of an organizational chart that incorporates these ideas for product-line management is shown in Figure 9–1. This may be compared with an organizational chart for a matrix structure, as presented in Figure 9–2.

An important facilitator of the product-line organizational structure is the product manager. As noted previously, product-line management can apply to either marketing and pricing or cost control. If it involves marketing and pricing, the product-line managers should report to the marketing executive and will have limited authority. If it involves cost control, the product-line manager has increased responsibilities, but not necessarily more authority. Product-line managers link products

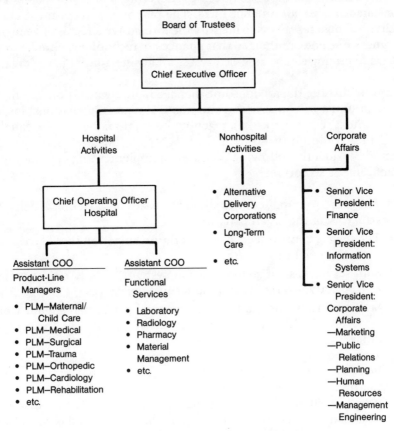

**Figure 9–1** Example of a Product-Line Management Organization Chart

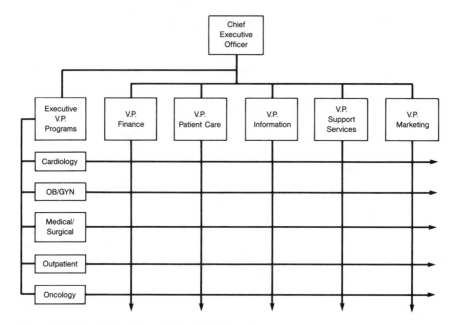

**Figure 9–2** Health Care Organization Matrix Structure

and functions. They must command respect and be problem solvers as well as key marketing advocates for their products. Their job is a difficult one to fill.

As noted, the concept of product-line management, while more easily implemented in the teaching hospital, has equal applicability to community hospitals. Yet the relevant roles and responsibilities may be significantly different in a community hospital, particularly in a rural hospital, compared with those in a teaching hospital. For example, in a community hospital, the product-line managers may be assistant administrators with three or four product lines. The assistant administrator might develop the business plans and manage the marketing of the product-line managers. In this scenario, top management would have both functional and product-line responsibilities.

**An Action Plan for Product-Line Management**

Once the top management of a hospital begins to implement a product-line management philosophy, certain steps should be followed to develop the requisite product-line management organization and delivery system. The following are six key steps in the action plan:

1.  Inform top management, physicians, and board of trustees of the
    projected product-line management philosophy and determine
    whether the organization needs a product-line management struc-
    ture to succeed in the present or anticipated health care environ-
    ment.
2.  Determine the product lines (business units) of the organization.
    The business units should be mutually exclusive and clinically
    identifiable within and outside the organization.
3.  Identify organizational responsibilities from both functional and
    product-line perspectives.
4.  Develop a new product-line planning and budgeting process.
    Review existing decision support systems and assess their ability
    to serve that process.
5.  Communicate information about the organizational structure
    from the top through middle-management levels. Convert the
    relevant managers to the product-line management philosophy,
    emphasizing the accountability, budgeting, and planning func-
    tions based on a product-line organizational structure.
6.  Reassess the product-line organization, business-unit philoso-
    phies, and responsibility-reporting relationships on a defined peri-
    odic basis.

In conjunction with these action steps, the hospital should consider
the impact of the product-line management organization in terms of its
overall delivery approach. An inconsistent responsibility-reporting system will result in an inefficient delivery of services. Product-line management is not for every hospital, but it is becoming increasingly
important as a basis for survival in the competitive environment of the
late 1980s.

It should be remembered that product-line management is not an
accounting function but rather an organizational function. It is highly
dependent on the definition of product lines and the number of product
lines to be managed. Because it relates to key decision makers, it is as
much an art as a science.

A move to product-line management requires increased communication between the product business units and ancillary and service organizations, simply because a high percentage of product costs originate
from the latter organizations. And, because such a move must involve
both the organizational structure and the key resource managers, the
implementation should be a top-down, not a bottom-up process. In each
case, the rate and scope of the process must be balanced with the key
resource managers' abilities and willingness to make decisions.

## Performance-Based Compensation[2]

A major part of any organizational system is the implementation of a compensation plan that promotes the mission and goals of the organization. It should include an employee incentive plan designed to increase employee motivation, help the hospital retain good workers and attract top physicians and employees, and result in increased profitability to the organization. It should demonstrate to top and middle management employees that the hospital values and trusts them and regards them as an important part of the delivery team. This will result in a more satisfied employee and top management, and will ultimately lead to greater satisfaction at the patient level.

Various organizations have used different types of incentive approaches. Three points warrant specific attention when setting up an incentive-based compensation system:

1. The system must be formulated around the organizational strategic objectives and the management structure that is already in place.
2. The development of an overall compensation philosophy is essential in the establishment of an effective incentive program. With such a philosophy, the organization can articulate the desired degree of linkage between performance and reward, the desired degree of risk versus reward, and role of other compensation components (for example, base salary, long-term incentives, and benefits/perquisites).
3. The incentive program should be built on a competitive base salary program. Many organizations attempt to rectify noncompetitive salary programs by instituting an incentive plan. This only serves to demotivate executives. In this connection, implementation of the incentive system may require the help of an outside specialist, someone who can provide insights into the accounting, performance, and tax consequences of the plan.

In sum, an effective incentive plan is one in which an employee's incentive payment is related to the hospital's overall performance and development and, to the extent possible, to the individual employee's own contribution to the hospital's growth.

---

[2]The material in the following discussion of performance-based compensation has been adapted from "Incentive Plans That Fit" by R.M. Haddrill and J.E. Moyer, *Ernst & Whinney Ideas*, pp. 21–23, Ernst & Whinney, Fall/Winter 1986.

Incentive-based performance systems will vary based on the individual employee responsibilities. For example, a product-line manager's responsibility may include marketing a product line to HMOs and bringing on physicians within that product line. In contrast, a functional department manager may be more likely to base performance on efficiency of operations and interdepartmental relationships. In any case, ultimately, the performance rewards must promote the actions of top managers as a team, rather than as individuals. Therefore, the performance rewards should tie into the performance of the organization as well as the individual. For organizations that manage for-profit subsidiaries under a parent corporation, there may be ways of tying an employee's compensation to the performance of the for-profit venture. One way this can be done is to provide stock options to employees of the for-profit ventures.

There are other ways to provide incentives for performance that are not directly related to the employee. These include profit-sharing plans, deferred compensation plans, and specific investment opportunities. Again, these plans may require outside assistance in implementation, due to tax and other statutory requirements.

Whatever the nature of the incentive plan, it is paramount that it be understood by all employees. If they are confused about what the hospital is doing for them, neither the hospital nor the employee will derive full benefit from the plan.

## SUMMARY

A variety of organizational structures can be applied to meet a hospital's management objectives. The choice of the appropriate structure is often a result of an analysis of the collective thoughts and objectives of the hospital's top management and board of directors. By viewing the projected organizational structure within the context of a cost management philosophy, the hospital will be better able to clarify its needs and achieve its objectives.

**REFERENCES**

John Child, *Organization* (New York: Harper & Row, 1977), 10.

Richard L. Daft, *Organizational Theory and Design*, 2nd ed. (St. Paul: West Publishing Company, 1986), 213.

# chapter 10

# Managing with Cost Information

## INTRODUCTION

Over the last several years, developments in the health care industry have encouraged greater competition between health care providers. With this competition has come new threats and opportunities and a greater need for accurate, timely, and reliable information on which to base decisions. Much of this information—such as planning, profitability, and performance information for product (service) lines, physicians, payers, and employers—can now be obtained from a cost management system. However, in the process, each management level must be provided with its own appropriate information, so as not to be either overwhelmed or underinformed.

Whereas the previous chapters examined the process of cost management, this chapter addresses the uses of cost management information to monitor performance and support both strategic and operational decision making. The related issues are discussed under the headings of performance reporting, pricing, and planning and budgeting. In each section, we provide interpretations and examples of reports and processes to facilitate the reader's understanding.

## PERFORMANCE REPORTING

For many hospitals, performance reporting is the most important and valuable function of a cost management system. Performance reporting provides hospitals—or any organization, for that matter—with an enhanced ability to reduce and control costs and monitor profitability. By periodically comparing strategic and operational plans with actual results, managers are provided with measurements of their performance for the aspects of the organization they control.

The performance reporting function provides several benefits to hospitals:

- It helps focus attention on problem areas (management by exception) by explicitly determining why a variance occurred and objectively determining the magnitude of the problem. Because aberrant outcomes are reported soon after they arise, solutions toward problem resolution can be formulated quickly and effectively. Additionally, for problems affecting the delivery of services in multiple departments (locations)—such as problems in scheduling and delivering bedside procedures—the magnitude of performance deviations can be summed across departments (locations) and then reported to top management for evaluation and resolution. This not only improves delivery and productivity, it may also, by more efficiently focusing on patient problems, reduce the length of stay and resource consumption.

- By determining why a problem occurred, responsibility, as identified in the planning process, can be attributed to a particular individual, leading to a clearer identification and measurement of performance. This becomes critical when evaluating managers and staff, determining areas of management weakness, planning management training needs, and implementing incentive compensation programs.

- By providing valuable cost management information for both products and operations, the performance reporting function provides management with a base for trend analysis. Through the storage of data and results for multiple periods, trend analysis enables management to clarify and measure performance based on past patterns. It also enables management to assess the progress of implemented solutions and to assess their effectiveness. Specifically, trend analysis reporting for multiple periods permits management to identify negative or positive trends that may be present and to determine their persistence over time.

Performance reporting occurs at both product and departmental levels. It spans virtually all managerial levels and disciplines—physicians, product-line managers, department managers, and top management. Again, however, it is important to understand that performance reports are not an end in themselves; they serve merely as the focal point for further analysis and investigative action. By ascertaining the degree of variance—either positive or negative—management can make adjustments to eliminate undesirable performance and to encourage and reward performance in excess of expectations. The outcome is an enhanced ability to reduce and control costs.

## Product-Line Performance Reporting

### Cost Variances

A cost management system produces product performance reports to address the product-line and clinical management control objectives of the hospital. The identification and quantification of product performance is done through a series of variances. Each variance isolates and measures the impact that a single factor has on performance.

Assume, for example, that a reporting period has just ended and the hospital is now reviewing actual product-line performance against planned expectations. Without accurate cost information and a cost management system, the hospital would probably produce a simplistic net revenue report similar to that in Exhibit 10–1. Based on the information provided by that report, management might conclude that the product line is being well-managed, since net revenue is four percent above expectations. However, if the product line's costs were known, a more realistic indication of performance would be obtained.

Product-line performance reports are useful in explaining those factors that affect performance. The cost-related factors that the product-

**Exhibit 10–1** Example of a Product-Line Net Revenue Report

Memorial Hospital
Product-Line Net Revenue Report
Period Ending: December 31, 19XX

| | Net Revenue | | | |
|---|---|---|---|---|
| Product Description | Actual | Planned | Variance | % |
| . | . | . | . | . |
| . | . | . | . | . |
| . | . | . | . | . |
| 138 Cardiac arrhythmia and conduction disorders age > 69 and/or C.C. | $ 50,500 | $ 71,000 | ($20,500) | (29) |
| 139 Cardiac arrhythmia and conduction disorders age < 70 w/o C.C. | 62,600 | 82,800 | (20,200) | (24) |
| 140 Angina pectoris | 88,600 | 56,200 | 32,400 | 58 |
| . | . | . | . | . |
| . | . | . | . | . |
| . | . | . | . | . |
| Totals | $851,800 | $822,100 | $29,700 | 4 |

line performance reports focus on are volume, mix, and treatment. Additionally, since treatment variances may directly affect them, net revenues actually received compared with planned revenues are reported.

An example of a product-line performance variance report that incorporates relevant cost information is presented in Exhibit 10–2. This report represents the initial step in reviewing the performance of the product line and its individual products. When compared with the information in Exhibit 10–1, the product line's real performance can be seen to be dramatically below expectations (44 percent). This variance is due to volume, mix, and treatment factors. The cost management system produces variance reports for each of these factors, and the reports are distributed to product-line managers, physicians, and other hospital executives for review and a determination of how each factor influences the actual performance of the product line.

*Volume and Mix Variances*

The report in Exhibit 10–3 shows a product-line's volume and mix variances as they relate to the report presented in Exhibit 10–2. The

**Exhibit 10–2**  Example of a Product-Line Performance Variance Report, Including Relevant Cost Information

Memorial Hospital
Cardiology Services
Product-Line Profit Summary Report
Period Ending: December 31, 19XX

| Product Description | Actual | | | Planned | | | Profit Variance | |
|---|---|---|---|---|---|---|---|---|
| | Net Revenue | Costs¹ | Profit Margin | Net Revenue | Costs | Profit Margin | Amount | % |
| 138 Cardiac arrhythmia and conduction disorders age > 69 and/or C.C. | $ 50,500 | $ 31,815 | $18,685 | $ 71,000 | $ 47,320 | $ 23,680 | ($ 4,995) | (21) |
| 139 Cardiac arrhythmia and conduction disorders age < 70 w/o C.C. | 62,600 | 44,202 | 18,398 | 82,800 | 59,200 | 23,600 | (5,202) | (22) |
| 140 Angina pectoris | 88,600 | 90,076 | (1,476) | 56,200 | 58,630 | (2,430) | 954 | — |
| Totals | $851,800 | $769,000 | $82,800 | $822,100 | $675,400 | $146,700 | ($63,900) | (44) |

¹Actual treatment at standard costs

**Note:** Other pertinent reporting options include presenting information by physician or by payer.

**Exhibit 10–3** Example of a Product-Line Performance Report Showing Volume and Mix Variances

Memorial Hospital
Cardiology Services
Product-Line Volume and Mix Variance Report
Period Ending: December 31, 19XX

| Product Description | Activity—All Cases | | | | Planned Profit Per Case | Profit—All Cases | | | |
| --- | --- | --- | --- | --- | --- | --- | --- | --- | --- |
| | | | Variance | | | | | Variance | |
| | Actual | Planned | Amount | % | | Actual | Planned | Amount | % |
| ⋮ | ⋮ | ⋮ | ⋮ | ⋮ | ⋮ | ⋮ | ⋮ | ⋮ | ⋮ |
| 138 Cardiac arrhythmia and conduction disorders age > 69 and/or C.C. | 23 | 37 | (14) | (38) | $640 | $14,720 | $ 23,680 | ($8,960) | (38) |
| 139 Cardiac arrhythmia and conduction disorders age < 70 w/o C.C. | 31 | 40 | (9) | (23) | $590 | 18,290 | 23,600 | (5,310) | (23) |
| 140 Angina pectoris | 36 | 22 | 14 | 64 | ($110) | (3,960) | (2,420) | (1,540) | (64) |
| ⋮ | ⋮ | ⋮ | ⋮ | ⋮ | ⋮ | ⋮ | ⋮ | ⋮ | ⋮ |
| Totals | 271 | 256 | 15 | 6 | | $150,824 | $142,229 | $8,595 | (6) |

reason that product-line volume and mix variances are combined on a single report is that the volume and mix variances are interrelated and both are the responsibility of the product-line manager. For example, differences in the activities of individual products will affect both the product line's total volume and the proportional mix of individual products. The product-line manager is usually responsible for forecasting the total volume of the product line and the proportional volume of its individual products.

Variance dollar amounts are quantified using standard amounts. The reason for this is that performance reporting should focus on only one factor at a time, in order to pinpoint responsibility and indicate the impact each factor had on performance. The amount of fixed costs assigned to a product may vary, depending on several factors, such as the total number of procedures produced by the department or aberrant expenditures on discretionary fixed costs. In this situation, the cost management system will provide management with a clear delineation of responsibility and a more exact measurement of performance.

Variances in procedure unit costs are the responsibility of functional department managers and therefore should not influence the evaluation of performance of product-line managers or the product line. While functional variances can be assigned to procedures, and then up to a product-line level, the accuracy of the assignments will vary—possibly leading to misinterpretation of the product line's real performance.

What information does the volume and mix report in Exhibit 10–3 provide to management? First, the actual total volume for the product line is six percent above forecasted levels (15 divided by 256). However, a significant shift from several more profitable products (product numbers 138 and 139) to products with negative profitability (such as product number 140) has occurred. The overall effect of volume and mix differences like these is the conclusion that the mix of products has adversely affected the profitability performance of the product line, even though overall volumes exceeded expectations.

To further examine and pinpoint the causes of the product-line volume and mix variance, the same type of reports could be produced, using criteria that further subdivide the product line—such as by physician, by payer, or by a specific geographic area. Such reports would provide further insights into the causes of shifts in the volume and mix of products, making problem identification and resolution more effective. Table 10–1 presents a brief list of common causes of product-line volume and mix variances. After the appropriate volume and mix reports are reviewed and the causes of the variances evaluated, the appropriate

**Table 10–1**  Common Causes of Product-Line Volume and Mix
Variances

- Following the hospital's volume forecast, the opening or closing of a similar facility or product line by a competitor.
- The loss or acceptance of a significant third-party contract that was offered or was up for renewal during the year.
- Failure to recognize the changing health care needs of the community, leading to both unexpected volume and mix deviations.
- Unforeseen operational problems, such as a breakdown in vital equipment, that forces temporary changes in clinical treatment capabilities.
- A change in physician complement that may provide the hospital with additional specialists, thereby increasing volumes and mix intensity, or result in the loss of key physicians or specialists, thereby reducing volumes and mix intensity.
- The positive or negative results of marketing efforts undertaken by the hospital, overall or for a particular product line.

action plans should be formulated and executed and then subsequently monitored to check on their effectiveness.

*Treatment Variances*

Treatment variances also contribute to product-line performance deviations. The primary purpose of treatment variance reports is to provide physicians and clinical managers with information on how they perform in comparison with treatment guidelines. A secondary purpose is to examine the effect treatment variances have on the profitability of the product line. In practice, the actual types and amounts of procedures consumed by a given patient rarely coincide exactly with expectations. However, across large numbers of patients, there should be some consistency in treatment by a particular physician or physician group. This makes treatment variance reporting a valuable output of a cost management system. Examples of treatment variance reports are presented in Exhibits 10–4 and 10–5.

For clinical purposes, treatment variances are typically reported in terms of attending physician, physician group, or specialty. In each case, it should be emphasized that, while deviations from treatment guidelines—either positive or negative—provide a statistical and monetary measure of performance, they may offer little real insight regarding cost effectiveness and the quality of care. Therefore, treatment variances typically serve as educational tools to enable physicians to analyze and refine their practice patterns. Depending on the physicians' comfort level with standard treatment protocols as a basis of comparison, treat-

**Exhibit 10–4** Example of a Product Treatment Variance Report

Memorial Hospital
Product Treatment Variance Report
Period: December 1 to December 31, 19XX
No. Cases: 23

Product no.: DRG No. 138
Product Name: Cardiac arrhythmia and conduction disorders Age > 69 and/or C.C.

| Procedure Number/Name | Standard Unit Cost | Standard Procedure Usage | Actual Average Procedure Usage | Usage Variance | Cost Impact |
|---|---|---|---|---|---|
| Admissions/discharge procedures | | | | | |
| 100101 Admission—normal | $ 26.19 | 1 | 1 | — | — |
| 100109 Medical record processing | 42.12 | 1 | 1 | — | — |
| 100110 Billing | 32.70 | 1 | 1 | — | — |
| Nursing Procedures | | | | | |
| 300123 Nursing Care Level 1 | 43.13 | 1 | 1 | — | — |
| 300223 Nursing Care Level 2 | 69.85 | 2 | 1 | 1 | $69.85 |
| 300323 Nursing Care Level 3 | 83.42 | 2 | 1 | 1 | 88.42 |
| 300423 Nursing Care Level 4 | 115.39 | 2 | 3 | (1) | (115.39) |
| Day-of-stay procedures | | | | | |
| 200100 Normal meal | 8.79 | 13 | 18 | (5) | (43.95) |
| 200410 Laundry/linen—medical | 3.38 | 9 | 7 | 2 | 6.76 |
| 200950 Housekeeping—normal | 3.13 | 11 | 9 | 2 | 6.26 |
| Diagnostic and therapeutic procedures | | | | | |
| 800422 Chest x-ray pa/lat | 37.13 | 1 | 1 | — | — |
| 900123 Lab CBC | 2.85 | 1 | 2 | (1) | (2.85) |
| 900124 Lab electrolytes | 16.60 | 3 | 5 | (2) | (33.20) |
| 700011 EKG—bedside | 38.99 | 1 | 1 | — | — |
| 600910 IV therapy | 39.95 | 7 | 9 | (2) | (79.90) |
| Per-Case Cost Variance | | | | | ($104.00) |

**Exhibit 10–5**  Example of a Product Treatment Variance Summary Report

Memorial Hospital
Cardiology Services
Treatment Variance Summary Report
Period Ending: December 31, 19XX

| Product Description | Cost Per Case | | | Actual Cases | Cost—All Cases | | | |
|---|---|---|---|---|---|---|---|---|
| | Planned | Actual | Variance | | Planned | Actual | Variance | % |
| . . . | . . . | . . . | . . . | . . . | . . . | . . . | . . . | . . . |
| 138  Cardiac arrhythmia and conduction disorders age > 69 and/or C.C. | $1,279 | $1,383 | ($104) | 23 | $ 29,417 | $ 31,809 | ($ 2,392) | (8) |
| 139  Cardiac arrhythmia and conduction disorders age < 70 w/o C.C. | 1,480 | 1,425 | (55) | 31 | 45,880 | 44,175 | (1,705) | (4) |
| 140  Angina pectoris | 2,665 | 2,502 | (163) | 36 | 95,940 | 90,072 | (5,868) | (6) |
| . . . | . . . | . . . | . . . | . . . | . . . | . . . | . . . | . . . |
| Totals | | | | 271 | $714,898 | $755,969 | ($41,071) | (6) |

ment performance reporting may serve as the basis for incentive compensation plans for physicians. However, caution should be exercised here to ensure that the physician compensation programs meet payers' (for example, Medicare) requirements before implementation. Further investigations into tax codes (for private inurement issues) and quality assurance systems (to evaluate treatment outcomes) must be considered in the light of existing physician and management incentive compensation programs.

Treatment performance reports can provide extensive benefits for both the physicians and the hospital. For example, to ascertain the effectiveness of alternative technologies (for example, laser surgery), treatment variance reports from the cost management system can be used to stratify the cost effectiveness of resource consumption between new and traditional surgical technologies. Given accurate cost information, the financial impact of alternative treatment protocols—assuming identical outcomes—can be shown, placing the hospital at both a financial and a competitive advantage. Quality assurance programs can supplement the entire evaluation process to qualify the outcomes of alternative treatment protocols.

Individual physician performance can also be addressed through treatment variance reporting. By comparing treatment regimens with accepted norms, an objective assessment of physician performance can be determined and quantified. However, cost and quality are often inversely—not directly—related. For example, a physician who routinely performs a complicated procedure may be a lower-cost provider and produce favorable outcomes. Conversely, a lack of familiarity with a given procedure may result in poor cost performance and poor quality of care. The review of resource consumption concurrently occurs with a review of outcomes, enabling hospitals to assess objectively both cost effectiveness and the quality of treatment.

Educational programs—generally led by other physicians—regarding treatment activity can help to initiate more cost-effective and higher-quality treatment protocols. In this case, the cost management system can be used to monitor a physician's progress through its capability to produce treatment variance reporting on a periodic and trend basis. The ultimate clinical result of such improved information via the cost management system is more consistent, more cost-effective, and higher-quality treatment patterns—giving the hospital a better competitive advantage.

Treatment variance information can also be used to measure the effect that actual treatment practices have on a product line's performance. If the hospital uses product resource consumption profiles in the planning process, treatment variances will impact on the product line's performance, since actual resource consumption seldom coincides with expectations. Treatment variances may or may not be influenced by the product-line manager; for example, the product-line manager may or may not have responsibility for determining when upgrades in automation take place. The nature and degree of such influence will depend on the type and amount of control delegated to the product-line manager (see the discussion on organization strategies in the previous chapter).

If the product-line manager uses historical resource consumption profiles that are not reflective of current practice patterns—for example, profiles that have changed due to improved information being available to physicians—then planning, marketing, and profitability expectations will almost certainly be off target. The critical factor here is communication between the product-line manager and the physicians within the product line. If significant changes in practice patterns occur, they must be communicated to refine expectations about the product line. The improved information will generally lead to better decision making and better results. Thus, the use of treatment variance reports is circular in nature; the cost management system provides physicians with information to improve their performance, which subsequently impacts the planning, profitability, marketing, and overall performance of the product line. Some common causes of treatment variances are listed in Table 10–2.

Finally, by changing the amount of payment received, treatment variances may affect the product line's financial performance, as illustrated in Exhibit 10–6. Changes in payments are largely dependent on

---

**Table 10–2** Common Causes of Treatment Variances

- Unanticipated alternative treatment practices due to changing technology or medical techniques.
- A physician (group) that has not kept abreast of current medical techniques, when compared with other physicians (groups) within the same product line.
- A poorly defined product and product-line measure that produces treatment norms that lead to significant treatment variations.
- The availability of alternative treatment settings (for example, outpatient), leaving an unanticipated or disproportionate share of acutely ill or outlier inpatients being treated.
- A reduced capability to administer both clinical and cost-effective treatment, due to a continually deteriorating delivery mechanism (physical plant, skilled staff, etc.).
- The activity within an individual product or product line is too small to make comparisons of treatment valid, that is, a small sample size that statistically lends itself to significant deviations.

**Exhibit 10–6** Example of a Product-Line Net Revenue Report Showing Overall Financial Performance

Memorial Hospital
Cardiology Services
Product-Line Net Revenue Report
Period Ending: December 31, 19XX

| Product Description | Net Revenue Per Case | | | Actual Cases | Net Revenue All Cases | | |
|---|---|---|---|---|---|---|---|
| | Actual | Planned | Variance | | Actual | Planned | Variance |
| 138 Cardiac arrhythmia and conduction disorders age > 69 and/or C.C. | $2,196 | $1,919 | $277 | 23 | $ 50,508 | $ 44,137 | $ 6,371 |
| 139 Cardiac arrhythmia and conduction disorders age < 70 w/o C.C. | 2,019 | 2,215 | (196) | 31 | 62,589 | 68,665 | (6,076) |
| 140 Angina pectoris | 2,461 | 2,555 | (94) | 36 | 88,596 | 91,980 | (3,384) |
| . | . | . | . | . | . | . | . |
| . | . | . | . | . | . | . | . |
| . | . | . | . | . | . | . | . |
| Totals | | | | 271 | $851,800 | $870,228 | ($18,428) |

how third-party price schedules are structured—that is, on a per-diem basis, on a case type basis, and so on. For example, if payment is on a per-diem basis and the length of stay is shorter than anticipated, with the same or greater amounts of nonnursing services consumed, payments and subsequently profit margins would be reduced. Consequently, treatment variances should be reported by payer stratification as a basis for measuring their effect on payment variances. If renewal or adjustment clauses are included in payer arrangements, information concerning them may prove invaluable in adjusting price schedules to reduce financial loss or risk to the hospital.

A major problem that is typically encountered in reporting actual payment is the general unavailability of such payment information on a timely basis, due to constraints in billing/receivables/collection systems. Thus, variances attributable to different payment amounts might remain hidden for a considerable period of time, constraining the product-line manager's ability to act. Another complicating factor may arise when contracts are structured on a capitation basis. In such cases, the profitability figures will be available only after the contract has expired, especially if the patient is admitted multiple times during the coverage period. With such capitated contracts, the volume, mix, and treatment variances must be monitored closely because of the increased risk involved.

By combining the information from the variance reports we have described, a clear measurement and understanding of product-line performance can be attained. This information can then be communicated to board members to show how the hospital's product lines have performed. Exhibit 10–7 presents an example of a board-level product-line performance report.

**Departmental Performance Reporting**

A cost management system also produces performance reports at the departmental (functional) level. These reports can be used by management to monitor departmental costs in a more effective manner—leading to cost reduction and enhanced cost control. Like product performance reporting, departmental management performance is measured through a series of variances, with each variance focusing on a different factor that may have caused a deviation from targets. Departmental variance analysis is an important ongoing component in the organization's efforts to meet its cost management objectives. Also, significant departmental cost reduction opportunities often surface during the implementation of the cost management system.

**Exhibit 10–7** Example of a Board-Level Product-Line Performance Report

Memorial Hospital
Product-Line Performance Report
Period Ending: December 31, 19XX

| Product-Line Description | Profitability | | Variances | | | |
|---|---|---|---|---|---|---|
| | Actual | Planned | Volume and Mix | Treatment | Revenue | Total* |
| Ophthalmology | $133,916 | $102,313 | $21,605 | $19,698 | ($ 9,700) | $ 31,603 |
| Pediatrics | 74,810 | 51,878 | 15,209 | 12,961 | (5,238) | 22,932 |
| Cardiology services | 82,800 | 146,700 | (4,401) | (41,071) | (18,428) | (63,900) |
| . | . | . | . | . | . | . |
| . | . | . | . | . | . | . |
| Totals | $910,123 | $808,204 | $81,877 | $45,602 | ($25,560) | $101,919 |

*May include differences due to rounding

*The Standard-Setting and Procedure-Costing Basis*

In the standard-setting process, a thorough analysis of the efficiency and effectiveness of each department's operations is made. Once the standards are set, the documented inefficiencies can be quantified and previously hidden inefficiencies, such as excess clerical time, can be uncovered. Corrective actions—such as adjusting staffing levels, enhancing automation, improving production techniques, and improving scheduling patterns—can then be implemented to reduce costs and/or improve delivery. Finally, the performance monitoring capabilities of the cost management system are used to ascertain the progress and results of the cost-saving measures over time.

To minimize start-up efforts, some hospitals implement a top-down, relative value unit (RVU) based approach that allocates actual or budgeted costs to individual procedures. However, though such an approach may be useful in expediting pricing applications, it is not necessarily effective in reducing or controlling costs. Any top-down approach will sidestep the issue of determining which costs should be incurred in producing a department's outputs.

By using standards representing qualified expectations of resource consumption and cost, the productivity of each labor category in each department can be assessed during the implementation/start-up phase of the cost-determination process. This bottom-up approach provides a more accurate comparison of earned resource and cost requirements with actual consumption than more traditional productivity overviews. The resulting increased accuracy in turn provides greater reliability in identifying the magnitude of production and staffing problems. This can lead to such cost management and delivery improvement opportunities as altering staffing through the cross-training of personnel, altering work flows, or enhancing scheduling policies, procedures, and systems.

The identification and documentation of indirect departmental labor activities—such as supervision, training, and so on—during the procedural standard-setting process can also lead to cost reduction opportunities. For example, in periods of increasing demand for a particular service (for example, outpatient surgery), the number of supervisory as well as technical personnel typically increases. However, as competitors enter the marketplace or other services satisfy a portion of the demand, declining utilization often follows.

Current staffing levels often go unchallenged due to a lack of accurate available information. By isolating and identifying such indirect activities and comparing them with industry norms, an objective evaluation of their necessity and cost-effectiveness can be made. The result

is often an improvement in a key component of organizational resizing—a better balancing of workload and workforce levels at supervisory,
as well as technical levels.

The concurrent review of direct and indirect labor costs during procedural standard-setting and reasonableness testing of initial results
provides an amplification of cost reduction opportunities. Exhibit 10–8
and Figure 10–1 illustrate how this information may expose potential
areas of cost reduction.

Procedure costing also gives the hospital the information it needs to
seek certain services from outside organizations, that is, make-versus-
buy decisions. The reason a hospital may seek an outside supplier is that
it might thereby obtain a more competitive price (reduce costs to the

**Exhibit 10–8**  Example of a Departmental Hour and Cost
Reconciliation Report

Cost Center: Diagnostic Radiology

| | Labor Hours | | | |
| Account Classification | Earned Hours[1] | Actual Hours | Variance | % |
| --- | --- | --- | --- | --- |
| 100 Manager | 2,120 | 2,080 | 40 | 2 |
| 200 Technician | 24,340 | 30,186 | (5,846) | (24) |
| 300 Clerk | 5,340 | 7,348 | (2,008) | (38) |
| 400 Secretary | 2,336 | 2,241 | 95 | 4 |
| Totals | 34,136 | 41,855 | (7,719) | (23) |
| | Earned Dollars | Actual Dollars | Variance | % |
| | Supply/Other Dollars | | | |
| Supply/other | $291,456 | $297,660 | ($6,204) | (2) |
| | Capital Dollars | | | |
| Capital | $112,800 | $112,800 | $0 | 0 |

[1]Calculated by multiplying actual procedure volumes by their respective variable cost components and adding in fixed cost components.

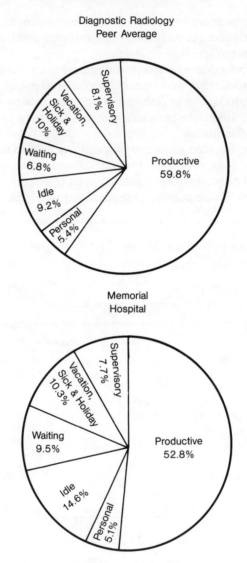

**Figure 10–1** Department-Level Comparison of Labor Components

hospital), improve delivery capabilities, or improve the quality of the service. The cost management system and the process of cost determination provides the basis for making such make-versus-buy decisions.

For example, suppose a hospital documents the operations of its dietary department and determines the costs of the services it provides and that, as a result of these efforts, it uncovers serious delivery problems, such as the fact that its food processing equipment is frequently breaking down and needs replacement. Moreover, the entire dietary area will have to undergo major renovations to accommodate the equipment changes.

Before a decision is reached regarding this kind of capital investment, the hospital should compare its current and projected dietary costs (including capital outlays) with prices from outside suppliers. If the outside supplier's price (the hospital's cost) is significantly less than the hospital's current or projected internal cost, the hospital should consider contracting for the required dietary services from the outside supplier. Other issues—such as overhead, union contracts, the hospital's lay-off policy, and overall personnel morale—may also have to be considered during the make-versus-buy decision process.

Another typical situation in which procedure costing may lead to a buy decision, but not necessarily for a full scope of services, involves the laboratory. Smaller and medium-sized hospitals can often purchase certain diagnostic laboratory procedures from external laboratories. By reducing the range of internal laboratory procedures to those of a more generic nature, the costs of low volume or sophisticated testing can be avoided, thereby often improving the quality of testing.

To further enhance the savings potential, the costing process should address the costs of the various departments, wherever possible, on some predetermined timetable. Experience indicates that there is a tendency to regard the costs of overhead departments as fixed in nature and therefore beyond objective challenge. Conversely, costs in patient care departments are regarded as variable in behavior and therefore subject to greater scrutiny. In fact, all departments' costs need to be managed effectively and consistently if the hospital is to meet its strategic and profitability objectives.

A final outcome of the procedure standard setting process is the hospitalwide review of procedure definitions in the charge master listing. Many hospitals do not have formal policies for auditing the charge master. The initiation of additions or deletions is typically the responsibility of department managers. Indeed, in many cases, alternative or new supplies or new technologies are adopted by a department for existing procedures without altering the charge master. For example, new and highly expensive anesthesia agents may be substituted for less costly agents, but only a single time-based charge may continue to be used in the department.

Depending on the magnitude of the cost components, it may be more appropriate to charge for several levels of treatments within a department—one for time and one for supplies. To the extent charge-based payers still exist, this operational improvement would generate additional (appropriate) revenues. Similar procedures would apply in the case of supply items, such as prosthetics, pacemakers, and catheters. In each case, better operational performance within the department and in the hospital as a whole could be realized.

*Periodic Variances*

In contrast to the general opportunities for cost reduction arising from the standard-setting and procedure-costing process in the implementation of the cost management system, ongoing performance reporting can provide department managers and their supervisors with the information needed to monitor and assess the financial results of day-to-day decisions. Historically, most hospitals have produced periodic variance reports. However, the content of these reports has usually been merely an expression of the difference between originally planned targets and actual results. Exhibit 10–9 represents a typical report of this type.

Unfortunately, it is difficult to draw valid conclusions from this type of report, since the reasons for a variance occurring remain hidden, making it difficult to initiate appropriate corrective actions. Additionally, this type of report can easily be misinterpreted, due to its inherent inability to separate responsibility. Finally, in the use of such a report, planned amounts are often derived without the benefit of knowing procedure level standard costs and having a forecast of case mix.

*Specific Ongoing Variances*

With a cost management system, a series of departmental variance reports can be produced to show why variances have occurred and who is accountable. For example, x-ray film costs could be at greater than planned levels due to more procedures being done, to prices for the film that were higher than anticipated, or to inefficient use of x-ray film. Each of these factors should be analyzed separately to see what the specific problem is and who is responsible for the actions that caused that problem. Table 10–3 illustrates how the most common types of departmental variances are calculated.

The types of variance reports commonly produced by hospital cost management systems are those for planning, efficiency (labor), rate, and spending variances. The other variances shown in Table 10–3—supply efficiency and rate variances—are generally not produced by the hospital cost management system. This is usually due to the fact that most hospitals' materials management systems are unable to supply the raw

**Exhibit 10–9** Example of a Departmental Periodic Variance Report

Memorial Hospital
Departmental Variance Report
Diagnostic Radiology
Period Ending: December 31, 19XX

| General Ledger Account | Current Period | | | | Year to Date | | | |
|---|---|---|---|---|---|---|---|---|
| | Planned | Actual | Variance | % | Planned | Actual | Variance | % |
| 100 Manager | $ 3,000 | $ 3,000 | $ 0 | 0 | $ 9,000 | $ 9,000 | $ 0 | 0 |
| 200 Technician | 17,400 | 23,200 | (5,800) | (33) | 63,300 | 82,400 | (19,100) | (30) |
| 300 Clerk | 2,800 | 3,400 | (600) | (21) | 8,400 | 10,100 | (1,700) | (20) |
| 600 Office supplies | 700 | 610 | 90 | 13 | 1,800 | 1,705 | 95 | 5 |
| 700 Film | 16,250 | 13,320 | 2,930 | 18 | 47,600 | 38,715 | 8,885 | 19 |
| 800 Developer | 2,010 | 1,750 | 260 | 13 | 5,490 | 4,700 | 790 | 14 |
| 1000 Magazines | 100 | 50 | 50 | 50 | 150 | 50 | 100 | 67 |
| 1100 Seminars | 1,400 | 0 | 1,400 | 100 | 1,400 | 1,400 | 0 | 0 |
| 1400 Rent | 2,000 | 2,000 | 0 | 0 | 6,000 | 6,000 | 0 | 0 |
| 1400 Leases | 2,300 | 2,300 | 0 | 0 | 6,900 | 4,900 | 2,000 | 29 |
| Totals | $47,960 | $49,630 | ($1,670) | (3) | $150,040 | $158,970 | ($ 8,930) | (6) |

*Note:* ( ) = Unfavorable

**Table 10–3** Departmental Variance Calculations

|  | Efficiency | Rate |
|---|---|---|
| Labor | Actual vs. earned hours | Actual vs. standard labor rate |
| Material | Actual vs. earned material Costed at standard costs | Actual vs. standard price Multiplied by actual volumes |

data required to produce materials-related variances (for example, number of items actually consumed by a department in a given reporting period).

The first step toward monitoring, controlling, and reducing departmental costs on an ongoing basis is to present each department's variances in a single report. The second step is to determine which variances are the cause for concern and then to request cost management variance reports that specifically delineate the calculations and the possible causes of the identified variances. To simplify this process, thresholds of significance should be defined in absolute dollar amounts and expressed as a percentage of total planned or earned amounts; this will enhance the user's ability to focus only on those items that are exceptional. The third step involves discussions with each manager who is accountable for the variance. Based on the outcome of these discussions and on careful further investigation, action plans for resolution of the identified problems can be formulated and implemented and then monitored to determine their effectiveness.

Exhibit 10–10 presents a variance report that provides a summary of the types of variances that an individual hospital department can incur. While this type of report is at a level of detail that is appropriate for the department manager, it is probably too detailed for other levels of management. Furthermore, product-line managers and top management need to assess the performance of all cost centers under their span of control. Exhibit 10–11 represents a cost management system report that provides a snapshot of the performance of multiple departments simultaneously or of the hospital as a whole.

For the department manager, the next step in the variance analysis process is to have the cost management system produce detailed reports on each departmental variance that is deemed to be significant. Examples of detailed variance reports for selected variances and a discussion of the ways managers use the information presented in each variance report are presented in the following sections.

**Exhibit 10–10** Example of an Individual Department Variance Summary Report

Memorial Hospital
Department Variance Summary Report
Diagnostic Radiology
For the Month Ending: December 31, 19XX

| | Costs | | Variances | | | | |
|---|---|---|---|---|---|---|---|
| General Ledger Account | Planned | Actual | Planning | Efficiency | Rate | Spending | Total |
| 100 Manager | $ 3,000 | $ 3,000 | $ 0 | $ 0 | $ 0 | $ 0 | $ 0 |
| 200 Technician | 17,400 | 23,200 | (100) | (3,900) | (1,800) | 0 | (5,800) |
| 300 Clerk | 2,800 | 3,400 | 240 | (740) | (100) | 0 | (600) |
| 600 Office supplies | 700 | 610 | (60) | 0 | 0 | 150 | 90 |
| 700 Film | 16,250 | 13,320 | 3,700 | (470) | (300) | 0 | 2,930 |
| 800 Developer | 2,010 | 1,750 | 290 | 0 | 0 | (30) | 260 |
| 1000 Magazines | 100 | 50 | | | | 50 | 50 |
| 1100 Seminars | 1,400 | 0 | | | | 1,400 | 1,400 |
| 1400 Rent | 2,000 | 2,000 | 0 | | | 0 | 0 |
| 1500 Leases | 2,300 | 2,300 | 0 | | | 0 | 0 |
| Totals | $47,960 | $49,630 | $4,070 | ($5,110) | ($2,200) | $1,570 | ($1,670) |

**Exhibit 10–11** Example of a Departmental Group Variance Report Summary

Memorial Hospital
Departmental Group Variance Report Summary
Diagnostic Ancillary Departments
For the Period Ending: December 31, 19XX

| Department Name | Costs | | Variances | | | | |
|---|---|---|---|---|---|---|---|
| | Planned | Actual | Planning | Efficiency | Rate | Spending | Total |
| **Diagnostic radiology** | | | | | | | |
| Current period | $ 47,960 | $ 49,630 | $ 4,070 | ($ 5,110) | ($2,200) | $ 1,570 | ($ 1,670) |
| Year to date | 150,040 | 158,970 | 2,270 | (12,141) | (2,387) | 3,328 | (8,930) |
| **Chemistry lab** | | | | | | | |
| Current period | 100,716 | 93,202 | 9,056 | 4,030 | (3,658) | (1,914) | 7,514 |
| Year to date | 302,113 | 281,655 | 17,677 | 2,099 | 1,005 | (323) | 20,458 |
| **Hematology lab** | | | | | | | |
| Current period | 59,950 | 61,216 | 102 | 398 | (79) | (1,687) | (1,266) |
| Year to date | 187,403 | 184,038 | 1,986 | 5,092 | 205 | (3,918) | 3,365 |
| **EKG** | | | | | | | |
| Current period | 20,155 | 26,039 | (983) | (2,956) | (1,945) | 0 | (5,884) |
| Year to date | 65,069 | 74,607 | 144 | (7,503) | (2,179) | 0 | (9,538) |
| . . . | . | . | . | . | . | . | . |
| **Totals** | | | | | | | |
| Current period | $ 465,033 | $ 486,213 | $11,410 | ($15,498) | ($4,951) | ($12,141) | ($21,180) |
| Year to date | $1,372,021 | $1,401,002 | $16,118 | ($36,129) | ($5,702) | ($ 3,268) | ($28,981) |

*Planning Variances*

The planning variance report in Exhibit 10–12 is similar in structure and interpretation to a volume and mix product report. It reflects the differences between the number and type of procedures that were expected and the number and type of procedures that were actually incurred for a given reporting period. Because planned and actual procedure activity levels rarely, if ever, coincide, planning variances can serve as important aids in understanding why a total departmental variance occurred.

All costs appearing in the planning variance report are standard costs extended by their respective planned and actual procedure volumes. In essence, the planning variance is a budget-to-budget comparison—with planned amounts reflecting the hospital's original budget and the standard costs as extended by actual volumes representing the earned budget. Earned budgets—on both a dollar and a statistical basis—are used in the calculation and reporting of efficiency variances. Thus, the calculations in earned budgets can lend themselves to many uses and applications by the cost management system.

Planning variance reports are normally produced at various levels of detail, in order to meet the hospital's reporting objectives for its various levels of management. In addition, related statistical and dollar reports can be produced by the cost management system to aid users in understanding the sources of the planning variances (for example, due to the loss of a series of outpatient procedural volumes). All fixed costs appearing on the planning variance report are the same, since changes in volume is the factor under review.

Accountability for departmental planning variances must be assigned to the managerial level that is responsible for developing the planned procedure activity. For example, if hospital executives are responsible for developing procedure volumes, the accountability and justification for the planning variances rests with them. If, in such cases, the hospital also decides to provide its department managers with the planning variance reports, it must be clearly understood that such distribution is for informational purposes only. In this case, the responsibility for the planning variances clearly rests at the executive level, where the decisions controlling procedure volume and mix projections—such as those involving product-line marketing plans—were made and the actions to achieve those projections were instituted.

If department managers develop their own procedure volume and mix projections, the accountability for any planning variance must rest with the individual department managers. In this case, hospital executives

**Exhibit 10–12** Example of a Departmental Planning Variance Report

Memorial Hospital
Departmental Planning Variance Report
Diagnostic Radiology
For the Period Ending: September 30, 19XX

| General Ledger Account | Current Period | | | | Year to Date | | | |
|---|---|---|---|---|---|---|---|---|
| | Standard Cost at Planned Volume | Standard Cost at Actual Volume | Variance | % | Standard Cost at Planned Volume | Standard Cost at Actual Volume | Variance | % |
| 100 Manager | $ 3,000 | $ 3,000 | $ 0 | 0 | $ 9,000 | $ 9,000 | $ 0 | 0 |
| 200 Technician | 17,400 | 17,500 | (100) | (1) | 63,300 | 68,420 | (5,120) | (8) |
| 300 Clerk | 2,800 | 2,560 | 240 | 9 | 8,400 | 8,170 | 230 | 3 |
| 600 Office supplies | 700 | 760 | (60) | (9) | 1,800 | 1,930 | (130) | (7) |
| 700 Film | 16,250 | 12,550 | 3,700 | 23 | 47,600 | 41,050 | 6,550 | 14 |
| 800 Developer | 2,010 | 1,720 | 290 | 14 | 5,490 | 4,750 | 740 | 13 |
| 1000 Magazines | 100 | 100 | 0 | 0 | 150 | 150 | 0 | 0 |
| 1100 Seminars | 1,400 | 1,400 | 0 | 0 | 1,400 | 1,400 | 0 | 0 |
| 1400 Rent | 2,000 | 2,000 | 0 | 0 | 6,000 | 6,000 | 0 | 0 |
| 1500 Leases | 2,300 | 2,300 | 0 | 0 | 6,900 | 6,900 | 0 | 0 |
| Total | $47,960 | $43,890 | $4,070 | 8 | $150,040 | $147,770 | $2,270 | 2 |

*Note:* ( ) = Underplanned amounts

should still receive the departmental planning variance reports, for their information and as a basis for initiating actions to require the department managers to explain why significant variances occurred and how the circumstances causing the variances will be remedied.

Under most circumstances, the causes of departmental planning variances can be traced back to product variances. For example, assume that a hospital has based its annual strategic budget plan on a certain volume and mix of products and that its departmental operational plan and standard product treatment profiles have been extended at appropriate volumes. Since each product requires a different resource consumption profile with a different mix of procedures, a shift in the planned volume and mix of products will cause a departmental planning variance, with greater or lesser amounts of certain types of procedures being consumed. If actual treatment protocols deviate from expectations, different types and amounts of procedures would be consumed, resulting in a departmental planning variance. In this case, by tracing product variance reports through the cost management system to departmental variance reports, a better understanding of cause and effect, responsibility, and problem resolution can be formed. Table 10–4 provides a brief listing of the typical causes of departmental planning variances.

*Efficiency Variances*

Efficiency variance reports are actually a means of measuring productivity and are thus very similar to productivity reports in content and purpose. Their purpose is the assessment of the effectiveness of managers in controlling labor resources and costs, as compared with pre-established targets and actual activity volumes. If a hospital has a cost

---

**Table 10–4** Common Causes of Departmental Planning Variances

- Unanticipated product volume and mix variances, possibly due to marketing programs or the availability (or unavailability) of physicians.
- Treatment variances due to atypical physician behavior or poorly defined treatment standards from which departmental volumes were forecasted.
- A change in the type and volume of predominantly outpatient procedures, due to competition (for example, in diagnostic laboratory services) or an increased (or reduced) need for outpatient services.
- A poorly defined methodology for forecasting product—and subsequently procedure—demand, such as that forecast by overall hospital discharges, days, or visits.
- Changes in the department's production process that may change the type and volume of the procedures being produced (for example, the replacement of equipment or services offered via a new technology).

management system, it is generally unnecessary for it also to have a separate productivity monitoring system. In fact, if their respective results are different for the same reporting period, it may be detrimental to have two separate systems producing virtually the same type of report. This would happen, for example, if the bases for labor standards within the two systems were based on different assumptions.

**Labor Efficiency Variances.** Labor efficiency variances measure the differences between the quantity of labor hours actually consumed and what should have been consumed (earned labor hours) given the level of output actually realized. An example of a labor efficiency report is shown in Exhibit 10–13. Labor efficiency trend analysis reports are utilized extensively to ascertain the progress of staffing changes resulting from focused productivity studies or inappropriate staffing levels identified during the initial implementation or ongoing use of the cost management system.

Accountability for labor efficiency variances rests with the hospital's department managers, since they make the decisions that control the direct resource consumption in day-to-day operations. Their reports on labor efficiency variances provide vital information to top management for use in evaluating the performance of department managers and in controlling costs. Top management also uses labor efficiency reports to adjust staffing levels in times of declining activity or when wage negotiations are anticipated. Thus, these reports should be prepared in both summary and detail form to meet the needs of the various levels of management.

If both standard and actual labor hours and rates are captured by skill level, the labor efficiency variances may be reported by skill level within a department. The reporting of labor efficiency variances by skill level can lead to a better understanding and analysis of a department's productivity and efficiency. This may result in staff reductions in areas exhibiting significant excess staff for actual workloads and, thus, in reduced hospital costs with consistent delivery capability.

Labor efficiency variance reports also can serve as a signal to update procedure standards. For example, if a department's overall efficiency or efficiency within a skill level is near or above 100 percent for a number of periods, there may be a problem with the standards or in the reporting process (for example, double counting of volume). In this case, procedure standards should be revised as necessary to bring efficiency reporting into line and to maintain the quality and integrity of cost information for pricing and planning applications. Table 10–5 lists some common causes of labor efficiency variances.

**Exhibit 10–13** Example of a Labor Efficiency Variance Report

Departmental Labor Efficiency Variance Report
Diagnostic Radiology
For the Period Ending: December 31, 19XX

| General Ledger Account | Current Period | | | | Year to Date | | | |
|---|---|---|---|---|---|---|---|---|
| | Standard FTEs at Actual Volumes | Actual FTEs at Actual Volumes | Variance | Efficiency Percentage | Standard FTEs at Actual Volumes | Actual FTEs at Actual Volumes | Variance | Efficiency Percentage |
| 100 Manager | 1.0 | 1.0 | 0.0 | 100 | 1.0 | 1.0 | 0.0 | 0 |
| 200 Technician | 10.2 | 12.4 | (2.2) | 82 | 13.7 | 15.9 | (2.2) | 86 |
| 300 Clerk | 2.5 | 3.5 | (1.0) | 71 | 2.7 | 3.6 | (0.9) | 75 |
| Totals | 13.7 | 16.9 | (3.2) | 81 | 17.4 | 20.5 | (3.1) | 85 |

**Table 10–5** Common Causes of Departmental Labor Efficiency
Variances

- Inefficiency caused basically by overstaffing the department due to managerial
  ineffectiveness.
- Standards inaccurately set with respect to variable time or time that is fixed in relation
  to volume (for example, supervisory time).
- Unanticipated changes in the department's production process, such as:

  —implementation of improved scheduling systems, resulting in fewer delays
  —cross-training of personnel, reducing idle time
  —equipment/automation changes, such as frequent breakdowns or upgrades to more
  efficient equipment
  —changes in the education or skill level of staff

- Unexpectedly slow learning curve or start-up time for a major program the hospital is
  marketing.

---

**Supply Item Variances.** Major supply item variances are captured at
the product level as treatment variances. Normally, supply items are
reported as charge items in the billing system (for example, artificial
kidney or prosthesis). However, supply items consumed in the production of a procedure are reported under efficiency variances. Supply
efficiency variances are measured using the same methodology as that
for labor efficiency variances. However, most hospitals choose not to
calculate and report such variances, since actual supply item usage by
department on an item-by-item basis is generally not captured. In addition, the cost of capturing all the required supply efficiency variance
data elements typically exceeds the resulting benefits. However, as
materials management technology becomes more sophisticated, the
calculation of supply efficiency variances will probably become more
common.

*Rate Variances*

A rate variance is another type of variance typically reported for cost
control purposes at the departmental level. Rate variances measure the
differences between standard labor and materials unit prices and what
was actually paid. To quantify the cumulative effect of rate variances,
unit price differences are extended by the total quantity of labor hours
and materials items actually used, to produce the reporting period's
total actual volume and mix of procedures.

Most hospitals calculate rate variances only for labor, since labor
represents the majority of a hospital's variable costs and is easily

obtained (from the payroll system). An example of a labor rate variance report is presented in Exhibit 10–14. Supply rates are more difficult to obtain on an actual basis, due to limitations in most materials management systems. A compounding complication in material rate variance calculations is the hundreds of items used throughout the hospital, with the majority of them having a unit cost of less than $5 and with total annual expenditures of less than $100,000. This makes the cost benefit of producing such reports of questionable value.

The line of responsibility for labor rate variances can take several different paths. For example, if the variances are due to changes that are a result of the hospital's human resources department or because of action at the executive level (for example, contract negotiations), department managers should not be held accountable for them. Rather, top management should be held accountable for the variances, with department managers receiving relevant labor rate variance reports for informational purposes only. However, if a department manager has the ability to influence the department's employees' wage rates (for exam-

**Exhibit 10–14**  Example of a Departmental Labor Rate Variance Report

Departmental Labor Rate Variance Report
Diagnostic Radiology
For the Period Ending: December 31, 19XX

| General Ledger Account | Planned | Actual | Variance | Actual Hours Incurred | Variance |
|---|---|---|---|---|---|
| | | *Hourly Rate* | | | |
| | | | *Current Period* | | |
| 100 Manager | $17.34 | $17.34 | $   0 | 173 | $    0 |
| 200 Technician | 9.63 | 10.75 | (1.12) | 2,143 | (2,400) |
| 300 Clerk | 5.85 | 5.52 | .33 | 606 | 200 |
| Total | | | | | ($2,200) |
| | | | *Year-to-Date* | | |
| 100 Manager | $17.34 | $17.34 | $  0 | 519 | $    0 |
| 200 Technician | 9.63 | 10.01 | (.38) | 8,232 | (3,128) |
| 300 Clerk | 5.85 | 5.45 | .40 | 1,853 | 741 |
| Total | | | | | ($2,387) |

ple, through merit increases), a sharing of the responsibility for the labor rate variances with top management is appropriate.

The overall value of labor rate variance information to the hospital stems from the enhanced ability it provides to monitor labor costs and to provide guidance for the direction and substance of future wage plans. Some common causes of labor rate variances are listed in Table 10–6.

While supply rate variances are normally an issue requiring future adjustment, they still may represent an important current cost element that the hospital must control. For example, if a major supply item, such as a hip joint, is continually fluctuating in cost and the fluctuations are significant, the cost management system can alert department managers to this fact so they can update procedure costs or investigate alternative vendors. The benefit derived from the alerting information is therefore twofold. First, procedure costs can be maintained more accurately, thereby making product pricing and profitability determination and monitoring more accurate. Second, if alternative vendors with lower prices are discovered, costs to the hospital can be reduced. Without a system to monitor and communicate this type of information, the hospital may be placed in a competitive disadvantage or be making strategic decisions with misinformation. If supply rate variances are to be reported, it is generally recommended that they be calculated only for those items that are significant in *both* usage and unit price, in order to maximize the return on effort and to expedite processing and maintenance time.

The accountability for supply rate variances depends on which managerial unit of the hospital, the purchasing department or the functional department, controls the purchase price and vendor of materials. If the responsibility for the variances belongs with purchasing, functional department managers may receive material rate variance reports, but for informational purposes only. Top management should receive the

---

**Table 10–6** Common Causes of Labor Rate Variances

- Unforeseen changes in inflation that cause the hospital to raise, lower, or postpone wage increases incongruously to planned levels.
- Lay-offs (or turnover) of personnel with less (or more) seniority, resulting in a staffing mix of higher (or lower) paid personnel.
- Personnel working a significant amount of overtime that was not budgeted or otherwise anticipated (this should be interpreted as reflecting an increased overall departmental efficiency if increased volume caused the overtime).
- Replacing or adding new personnel at rates that are significantly different than those for existing personnel, due to an oversupply or shortage of qualified personnel.

material rate variance reports to assist them in analyzing the performance of purchasing personnel and functional department managers. Also, if they regularly influence the use of more expensive brand name supplies, physicians may be added to the distribution list.

## Spending Variances

A spending variance is another departmental variance that is typically reported by a cost management system. A spending variance represents the quantitative difference between planned and actual expenditures for fixed nonsalary costs. Spending variances inform management of levels of spending that are inconsistent with strategic or operational plans. By tracing the accountability for and the cause of such variances, corrective actions or rewards can be formulated.

For example, if a hospital plans to lease a lithotripter on January 1, but, due to a delay in remodeling the physical area for the lithotripter, the starting date for the lease is delayed until April 1, a favorable spending variance under the lease general ledger account for the relevant department would be recorded. This example suggests that the exact responsibility for spending variances may be difficult to determine.

As a general guideline, capital-related spending variances should be regarded as the responsibility of senior-level management—top management or product-line managers—since they generally set the plan to determine when capital commitments should be made and what products will be offered, often involving a demand for a new technology. Spending variances relating to other items—such as education programs and professional dues—are the responsibility of the department manager and are incurred at each department manager's discretion. Three common causes of departmental spending variances are listed in Table 10–7.

## Summary Performance Reports

In order to present departmental performance results to the board of directors in a meaningful format, all of the departmental performance

---

**Table 10–7** Common Causes of Departmental Spending Variances

- Placing an asset into service or retiring an asset before its scheduled timetable stipulates.
- Spending a different amount than planned for equipment or other items (for example, education seminars) or increasing the number of or the types of activities for departmental personnel (for example, education seminars, professional societies).
- Using an inadequate methodology to plan capital and other fixed types of expenditures.

reports described above should be summarized in a single report. This report may be prepared in various formats, depending on how the hospital is organized and what management wants to report when explaining performance results. For example, the hospital could report all nursing units together, all therapeutic ancillary units together, and so on, if its reporting structures were organized in this way. Alternatively, the summary report could be formatted at a more detailed level. An example of one type of a summary board-level departmental performance report is provided in Exhibit 10–15.

## PRICING

For many hospitals, securing or maintaining market position requires bidding competitively to provide services to defined populations. However, many hospitals prepare bids for services without the benefit of accurate cost information. The outcome of these information shortfalls is often significant cost misstatements or strategic difficulties—such as other insurers wanting similar discounts—leading in some cases to serious financial hardship. Subsequent corrective actions often result in raising prices for a smaller group of fee-for-service payers, causing the public to perceive the hospital as a "high-cost" provider. Clearly, to structure the prices of their products appropriately and to determine the risk and return on each competitive contract, hospitals need accurate, reliable, and timely cost information.

Pricing decisions based on accurate cost information enable the hospital to influence more precisely the utilization of its products and to understand the implications of related prices and risk levels. In addition, the monitoring of the results of accepted price schedules can provide insights to top management and the board of directors regarding the effectiveness of their pricing policies and decisions. While each competitive opportunity must stand on its own as to its priority, the proper interpretation and use of cost management information will provide the hospital with the means to achieve generally sound pricing policies. In short, effective pricing strategies require the right balance of activities and information, including cost information, to be successful.

### A Case Study: Memorial Hospital and Alpha Care HMO Cardiology Services

To demonstrate how a cost management system can support a hospital's pricing decision-making process, assume that Memorial Hospital

**Exhibit 10–15** Example of a Summary Board-Level Departmental Performance Report

Memorial Hospital
Summary Departmental Performance Report
For the Period Ending: December 31, 19XX

| | Cost | | | | Variances | | |
| Department Group | Planned | Actual | Planning | Efficiency | Rate | Spending | Total |
|---|---|---|---|---|---|---|---|
| Nursing | $2,325,041 | $2,181,316 | $39,037 | $34,959 | $27,919 | $41,810 | $143,725 |
| Nonclinical support | 217,033 | 203,508 | 6,108 | 9,877 | (470) | (2,090) | 13,425 |
| Diagnostic ancillary | 465,033 | 486,213 | 11,410 | (15,498) | (4,951) | (12,141) | (21,180) |
| . . . | . . | . . | . . | . . | . . | . . | . . |
| Totals | $5,703,819 | $5,811,612 | ($62,806) | $34,522 | ($31,611) | ($47,898) | ($107,793) |

receives a request from the Alpha Care HMO to submit a pricing schedule for cardiology services, with DRGs as the individual product measure. The first thing the hospital does is examine the population the HMO covers for the requested services and determine the proportion of that population to which the hospital is currently providing services. The hospital then asks for and obtains from Alpha Care current and future market share information for the proposed services. This quantifies the magnitude of both the opportunity and the risk involved.

Next, to obtain information regarding the number of Alpha Care patients for which the hospital currently provides cardiology services, Memorial's management accesses the cost management system's product reporting function. By analyzing this information in tandem with the market share data from Alpha Care, the absolute demand for cardiology services by Alpha Care enrollees is determined, and the hospital's relative share of those services is calculated. The resulting information may be organized in a demand analysis report format, as shown in Exhibit 10–16. This shows that a significant opportunity to increase cardiology services exists, given the total potential demand (over 1,000 cases) and Memorial Hospital's current share (16 percent) of Alpha Care patients. Therefore, in this case, the competitive bidding situation presents both an opportunity and a risk—the opportunity to increase the hospital's market share, and the risk of losing the share it already has.

### Analysis of Profitability Factors

While activity measures provide some insights into opportunities and risks, Memorial Hospital also must evaluate cost, margin, and overall profitability factors when formulating its decision to pursue an opportunity, especially in developing its pricing strategy. For example, if variable costs for cardiology services are greater than current gross charges, attempting to add more volume for those services at or below current prices will result in greater losses. Conversely, if variable costs are substantially below current gross charges and excess bed capacity exists, increasing volume will contribute to overhead and increase profitability.

In our example, gross profitability and margin information for each product covered by Alpha Care's request is obtained from Memorial's cost management system for analysis. The resulting cost, margin, and profitability data are summarized in a product-line gross margin and profitability report, as shown in Exhibit 10–17. Several key insights can be gained from this report. For example, the hospital has a substantial

**Exhibit 10–16** Demand Analysis Report of Alpha Care HMO
Cardiology Services

Memorial Hospital
Demand Analysis Report
Alpha Care HMO Cardiology Services
for Fiscal 19XX

| | *HMO Enrollees' Cardiology Services Demand* | | |
| Product Description | Total | Current Hospital Cases | Current Hospital Share |
|---|---|---|---|
| 138 Cardiac arrhythmia and conduction disorders age > 69 and/or C.C. | 95 | 16 | 17% |
| 139 Cardiac arrhythmia and conduction disorders age < 70 w/o C.C. | 82 | 21 | 26% |
| 140 Angina pectoris | 102 | 15 | 15% |
| . | . | . | . |
| . | . | . | . |
| . | . | . | . |
| Totals | 1,002 | 156 | 16% |

total margin and a moderate profitability for its entire cardiology service product line. Therefore, additional volumes of these cases—if added in the same mix—should increase the hospital's operating margin. Conversely, the loss of a significant portion of current cardiology service volumes may result in lower profits for the hospital.

Using this information, the profitability of the HMO cardiology services can be calculated at various volume levels, and the breakeven point (zero profitability) can be located. Memorial's management can compare this information with its Alpha Care activity assumptions to determine the feasibility of reaching a profitable level of activity and to structure its price schedule, based on certain activity thresholds.

Initially, the calculation of profitability and the breakeven point should use existing historical cost (actual treatment at standard costs) and revenue data as a basis. This provides as a starting point an audit trail of reliable information. Therefore, in our example, Memorial Hos-

**Exhibit 10–17**   Product-Line Gross Margin and Profitability Report Based on Alpha Care HMO Bid

Memorial Hospital
Cardiology Services
Gross Margin and Profitability Report
from October 1, 19XX through September 30, 19XX

| | Per Case | | | | | | Totals* | |
| Product Description | Gross Revenue | Variable Cost | Gross Margin | Fixed Cost | Gain (Loss) | Total Cases | Gross Margin | Gain (Loss) |
|---|---|---|---|---|---|---|---|---|
| 138 Cardiac arrhythmia and conduction disorders age > 69 and/or C.C. | $2,312 | $1,134 | $1,178 | $640 | $538 | 85 | $100,130 | $45,730 |
| 139 Cardiac arrhythmia and conduction disorders age < 70 w/o C.C. | 2,058 | 1,318 | 740 | 667 | 73 | 150 | 111,000 | 10,950 |
| 140 Angina pectoris | 1,904 | 1,526 | 378 | 519 | (141) | 105 | 39,690 | (14,805) |
| . . . | . . . | . . . | . . . | . . . | . . . | . . . | . . . | . . . |
| Average/Totals | $2,414 | $1,888 | $ 526 | $421 | $105 | 815 | $429,000 | $85,250 |

*Note:* Other pertinent reporting options include presenting information by payer, by employer, or by physician.
*Totals may include differences due to rounding.

pital uses the following cost management information: Revenue per case is at gross charges of $2,414, variable costs per case are $1,888, and fixed costs are represented by Alpha Care's current share of $65,676 ($421 per case × 156 cases). Incremental activity assumptions are applied against these historical data to enable the hospital to calculate the relevant profitability levels. The hospital's cardiology services profitability calculations at various levels of activity are shown in Exhibit 10–18.

The breakeven point is calculated by applying the above data in the following formula:

Revenue per case × Number of cases = [(Variable cost per case + Profit per case) × Number of cases] + Fixed costs

$2,414 × Breakeven units = [(1,888 + 0) × Breakeven units] + $65,676

$2,414 × Breakeven units = $1,888 × Breakeven units + $65,676

$526 × Breakeven units = $65,676

Breakeven units = 125

---

**Exhibit 10–18**  Profitability Analysis of Alpha Care HMO Cardiology Services

|  | Memorial Hospital | | | | |
|--|--|--|--|--|--|
|  | Profitability Analysis at Alternative Volume Levels | | | | |
|  | Alpha Care HMO Cardiology Services | | | | |
| Volume | Variable Costs | Fixed Costs | Total Costs | Gross Revenue | Profit (Loss) |
| 75 | $141,600 | $65,676 | $207,276 | $181,050 | ($ 26,226) |
| 100 | 188,800 | 65,676 | 254,476 | 241,400 | (13,076) |
| 125 | 236,000 | 65,676 | 301,676 | 301,750 | 74 |
| 150 | 283,200 | 65,676 | 348,876 | 362,100 | 13,224 |
| 175 | 330,400 | 65,676 | 396,076 | 422,450 | 26,374 |
| 200 | 377,600 | 65,676 | 443,276 | 482,800 | 39,524 |
| 225 | 424,800 | 65,676 | 490,476 | 543,150 | 52,674 |
| 250 | 472,000 | 65,676 | 537,676 | 603,500 | 65,824 |
| 275 | 519,200 | 65,676 | 584,876 | 663,850 | 78,974 |
| 300 | 566,400 | 65,676 | 632,076 | 724,200 | 92,124 |
| 325 | 613,600 | 65,676 | 679,276 | 784,550 | 105,274 |
| 350 | 660,800 | 65,676 | 726,476 | 844,900 | 118,424 |
| 400 | 755,200 | 65,676 | 820,876 | 965,600 | 144,724 |

Because the breakeven point of 125 cases represents the level of activity at which total revenue equals total costs, the profit per case is zero. Volumes above 125 cases will produce a profit, based on the hospital's assumptions of revenue, variable, and fixed costs.

The same breakeven point and profitability data can be expressed graphically to provide Memorial's management with a snapshot of profitability along an activity continuum. The resulting profitability and breakeven graph is shown in Figure 10–2.

## Structuring the Price Schedule

Memorial Hospital is now in a position to begin structuring its price schedule. Realizing the prices it submits to Alpha Care may have to be discounted, the hospital must review these key components:

- the number of expected cases
- changes in variable costs
- changes in fixed costs

Various factors may affect the number of cases Memorial Hospital expects to receive under the Alpha Care contract. These factors include the number of competitors who are offering similar services and from whom Alpha Care also is soliciting pricing schedules; exclusivity or guarantee covenants (for example, three hospitals may be selected, with each receiving one-third of the total volume); the availability of physicians who are contracting with Alpha Care and who also have admitting privileges at Memorial Hospital; and the projected demand for cardiology services over a period of years, for Alpha Care and for the service area in general.

Each of these factors must be analyzed by Memorial's top management, product-line managers, and physicians (where appropriate) to determine the probability of achieving selected activity levels. In our example, assume that several hospitals are competing for the contract and that there are no exclusivity or guarantee covenants. Based on an analysis of the above activity factors, Memorial's management determines that the lower and upper volume limits for the HMO contract are 150 and 300 cases, respectively. Management must now determine the probability of achieving each activity increment (25-case increments) within the expected volume range. A recapitulation of the relevant data is presented in an activity forecast analysis chart, as shown in Exhibit 10–19.

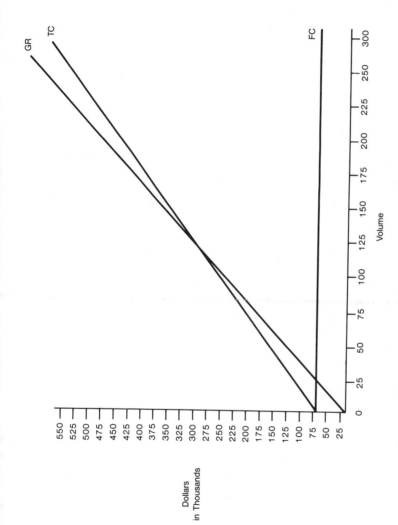

**Figure 10–2** Memorial Hospital Breakeven Chart for Alpha Care HMO Cardiology Services

*Note:* GR = gross revenue, TC = total costs, FC = fixed costs.

**Exhibit 10–19**  Activity Forecast Analysis Chart for Alpha Care HMO
Cardiology Services

| | Memorial Hospital | Alpha Care HMO Cardiology Services | | |
|---|---|---|---|---|
| | | Activity Forecast Analysis Chart | | |
| Incremental Activity Level | Probability of Achievement | Expected Incremental Activity | Base Activity Level | Total Expected Activity |
| First 25 | 90% | 23 | 150 | 173 |
| Second 25 | 75% | 41 | 150 | 191 |
| Third 25 | 55% | 54 | 150 | 204 |
| Fourth 25 | 40% | 64 | 150 | 214 |
| Fifth 25 | 30% | 72 | 150 | 222 |
| Sixth 25 | 25% | 78 | 150 | 228 |

It appears from this chart that Memorial Hospital cannot realistically expect more than about 228 cardiology service cases from Alpha Care, given the hospital's activity probability assumptions. This figure, together with the breakeven point, becomes the basis for determining benchmark activity levels when structuring the price schedule. This does not mean that the hospital cannot attempt to influence volume by further discounting, once certain activity levels are reached. For example, in an attempt to increase activity above expected levels or to encourage activity to realize at least its breakeven point, the hospital may offer deeper discounts for those cases in excess of 250 cases.

Variable and fixed cost components also need to be reexamined, based on the age and integrity of the cost data and the duration of the contract. For example, if the Alpha Care contract is for multiple years, costs will need to be trended forward, based on inflation assumptions. In this way, price schedules can be adjusted to reflect changes in cost over time and to maintain expected profitability levels. Most cost management systems have the capability to process various levels of inflation. For purposes of our example, we will assume that the Alpha Care contract is for one year only and that inflation is zero.

With the above assumptions of activity and cost components finalized, Memorial's management can now calculate the contribution and profitability of the anticipated 228 cardiology services cases, based on gross charges. This calculation produces a margin of $119,928 and an overall profitability of $54,252.

## Determining Profitability Requirements

The next task is to determine the profitability (return) requirements for the Alpha Care bid. There are several ways the hospital may determine its profitability level, and subsequently its prices, for the bid. For instance, the hospital may discount its services by a flat percentage, it may determine a certain contribution percentage above variable costs, or it may build in a flat dollar amount of return. Each hospital must establish its own pricing policy to apply to competitive situations. This is generally the responsibility of top management. In our example, we shall assume that Memorial Hospital desires a return of five percent over variable costs, in addition to the $65,676 of fixed costs already identified for recovery. Based on these assumptions, overall revenue of $517,572 is required for the forecasted 228 case volume. The relevant calculations are shown in Exhibit 10–20.

Memorial Hospital translates the required revenue into a discount percentage that is applied back to each case type (DRG in this instance). The discount percentage to be applied is calculated by dividing the required revenue of $517,572 by gross revenue for the 228 cases, $550,392 (228 × $2,414). The result, 94 percent, indicates a discount percentage of six percent. This percentage is applied back to each DRG to determine its particular revenue requirements. For example, the price for DRG No. 138 is $2,220 (94 percent of gross charges of $2,312).

Memorial's management may adjust the discount upward or downward, based on its perception of competition and risk. For example, if

---

**Exhibit 10–20**  Calculation of Required Revenue from Alpha Care
HMO Cardiology Services

| | |
|---|---:|
| Variable costs per case | $1,888 |
| 5 percent return | + $94 |
| Total | $1,982 |
| Forecasted cases | × 228 |
| Total | $451,896 |
| Fixed costs | + $65,676 |
| Total required revenue | $517,572 |

the hospital were to lose the Alpha Care contract, cardiology services volume from other payers may decline, due to physicians admitting all of their patients—for personal convenience reasons—to the hospital holding the Alpha Care contract. Also, the loss of market share in one program may affect other programs, based on physician and consumer perceptions of the hospital, for example, perceptions that the lost business is the result of high cost or a lower quality of care.

Another possibility in structuring Memorial's price schedule is to offer further discounts to Alpha Care HMO if activity exceeds a certain threshold. There are two key factors to consider when offering additional discounts above a certain threshold of activity. The first is the activity thresholds themselves; the second is the hospital's marginal costs. For example, even though total Alpha Care HMO cardiology service activity is estimated to be 228, the hospital may want to encourage business even at the base levels by placing its initial additional discount threshold at 200 cases. Multiple thresholds may be defined to encourage the HMO to send more of its cardiology patients to the hospital.

### Identification of Marginal Costs

Marginal costs are related to excess capacity in staff, space, and equipment. For example, if adequate staff and equipment exist, anticipated marginal costs in Memorial Hospital's cardiac catheterization department may be only the cost of the supplies actually consumed. However, if an influx of patients substantially above current volume levels occurs—presumably from the Alpha Care contract—additional staffing may be necessary. This new staffing may not necessarily be prorated for each additional patient. Rather, one or several full-time people may have to be added to cover the increased workload. If patient volume increases occur intermittently, departments such as cardiac catheterization may still have to hire additional staff in response to an as-yet-unknown level of additional volume. Thus, the marginal costs comprise not only the additional direct supplies consumed, but also the cost of the additional staff.

The identification of possible capacity constraints requires specific cost management information. This includes a listing by cost center of the number and type of procedures required to serve alternative demand assumptions, translated into staffing and equipment utilization requirements. This information is used to investigate cost centers with excess or limited capacity to provide services. The resulting analysis allows management to determine margins and profit thresholds based on capacity findings and to evaluate the impact of workload volumes, given alternative demand assumptions. This, in turn, may affect the risk and prices ultimately contained in the price schedule.

## Analysis of Other Relevant Factors

Before finalizing the price schedule in our example, Memorial Hospital should analyze the impact outliers have on profitability and margins. Outlier information comes from the cost management system's cost determination function. The analysis of such information is particularly appropriate when structuring the price schedule to provide a "safety net" for those cases that exceed a certain level of cost, based on days, gross charges, or other criteria.

A cost management system can provide a hospital with information, but it cannot make judgments. Thus, though gained or lost volumes and marginal cost data are derived from information provided by the cost management system, they require management interpretation, due to the uncertainty and interrelationship of assumptions, to become the basis for decision making. For example, anticipated volumes by product line depend on many interrelated factors—level of exclusivity, volume level, guarantees, physician incentives, physician admitting privileges, and so on. Thus, although a cost management system is clearly an essential management tool, it requires competent and properly trained people to make its data effective.

Accordingly, apart from cost management information, other factors that often influence the structure and content of the price schedule must be examined. For example, a hospital that offers a comprehensive set of related services (for example, cardiology services, cardiac rehabilitation, and wellness programs) may leverage those services in its bid. This may be an extremely attractive offer for the HMO or employer, since a richer benefit package may then be offered to their enrollees through a single provider.

Other factors affecting the price schedule may be quality and location characteristics. For example, if two hospitals offer similar services but one is in a better location or has a higher perceived quality or a real relative quality, it will be more attractive to the HMO or employer. Given these advantages, the hospital may be less willing to discount, or it may require volume guarantees, because it knows that the HMO or employer needs its services to attract enrollees. In this case, the hospital is giving the HMO or employer an additional inducement by offering its enrollees a more attractive place to obtain medical treatment.

Another factor affecting the price schedule may be the effect of lost volume within a program, as it moves from one payer to other payers and physicians. The loss of volume in one program may create a "domino effect" of volume losses in other programs. Some may perceive something wrong with a provider that was denied a bid, for example, identifying the provider with low-quality, high-cost, inadequate medical staff, and so on. For these reasons, the hospital may need to "protect" its volumes in other programs. However, in this kind of situation, it should be remembered that the protection of volume cannot be achieved solely by discounting services.

### Determining the Price Scheduling Structure

Finally, the actual structure of the price schedule (per diem, per discharge, etc.) must be determined. The structure of the price schedule may be specified by the HMO or employer, or it may be left to the hospital's discretion. Some common forms of price schedule structures and their associated risks are outlined in Table 10–8.

If, in our example, Memorial Hospital were required to determine prices on a per diem basis, it would have to take several additional steps in structuring the price schedule in order to minimize its risk. These include determining the costs incurred on each day of stay for each product and structuring the price per diem in conjunction with those costs. A graphic display of day-by-day cost information for a specific product is presented in Figure 10–3.

By structuring its price schedule in this manner, Memorial Hospital protects its profitability position by receiving revenue in accordance with the incurrence of costs. Moreover, if length of stay is reduced, due to advancing medical techniques and technologies, the hospital will most likely avoid losing revenue in excess of costs and eroding the profitability of the contract. Typically, in order not to overburden the price schedule with a different price for each day—and thereby possibly also revealing the hospital's margins—only one or two prices per diem for each product are quoted on the pricing schedule. A per diem price schedule submitted by Memorial Hospital to the Alpha Care HMO for cardiology services is presented in Exhibit 10–21.

### Negotiating with the Contractor

After the price schedule is finalized and submitted, negotiations with the contractor often follow. Negotiated items may include prices, risk issues, volume guarantees, and other contractual terms. With the relevant cost management information available to negotiate prices, the

**Table 10–8** Common Price Schedule Structures and Associated Risks

| Structure | Risks |
| --- | --- |
| Reductions from gross charges | There is minimal risk to the hospital, but it often is coupled with minimal opportunity for increased volume. Risk is limited unless significant shifts in the mix of products occur. This may result in eroding margins if across-the-board discounts are applied to all patients. Hospitals also must monitor the types of procedures being consumed and take action if more costly (lower margin) procedures are consumed in greater-than-anticipated proportions. |
| Per diem | Risk may increase with increasing amounts in the type and/or level of routine care provided (unless separate special care unit rates are used) or in ancillary resources consumed per day. The hospital needs to monitor new physicians' activities and its departmental capacity limits. |
| Per case (e.g., DRG) | In addition to the per diem risks, the risk of changes in overall length of stay is introduced. Hospitals must monitor total patient resource consumption—routine, special care, and ancillary services—within a case type. Changes in the level of care being provided within a case type also must be monitored. For example, as more lens procedures are performed in an outpatient setting, the cost of treating (the more seriously ill) inpatients increases. Finally, hospitals must evaluate and understand outliers and resource consumption deviations in their case mix. |
| Per discharge | In addition to the per case type of risk, the hospital is exposed to changes in case mix (for example, changes in hospitalization patterns across products). Services provided to patients may shift as a result of demographic changes within the community or as a result of the hospital's strategic actions (for example, changing the composition of its medical staff). |
| Capitation | In addition to controlling the cost of care provided, as in each of the above scenarios, the hospital assumes the actuarial risk of quantity and quality of care that will be required by enrollees. New information requirements include demographic and claims experience. New programs (for example, outpatient surgery) may help reduce some risk if they are administered in a cost-effective manner. |

hospital is in a position of control and can avoid decisions that may place it in an adverse strategic or financial position. It is also able to determine quickly if it can discount further, and what the consequences of further discounts would be. As in structuring the price schedule, the types of information that are most critical in the negotiation process are the marginal costs of each product, the deviations in and parameters of resources consumed by each product, and the amount of volume to be gained or lost. However, this information is needed on a more timely

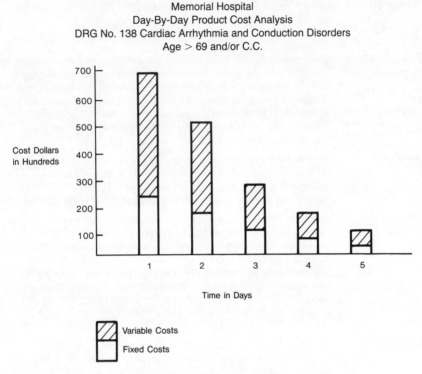

Figure 10–3 Day-by-Day Cost Figures for a Specific Product

and flexible basis in the negotiation stage, compared with the price structuring stage.

In the negotiation process, the price schedule and terms of the contract are either accepted or rejected by the contractor and hospital. If no agreement can be reached, the hospital may need to take action to reduce staff, develop a plan to recapture the lost business, or pursue other product lines more aggressively. If the price schedule is accepted, the contract's profitability and activity levels should be monitored to ensure that expectations are realized. The cost management system's product performance reporting function will provide the information needed to monitor the performance of the contracts.

### Procedure-Level Pricing

Cost management information is also essential for making pricing decisions at the procedure level. For example, a hospital may provide

**Exhibit 10–21**  Per Diem Price Schedule for Alpha Care HMO
Cardiology Services

| Product Description | Price Per Diem |
| --- | --- |
| 138 Cardiac arrhythmia and conduction disorders age > 69 and/or C.C. | $750 each day for two days, $240 each day thereafter |
| 139 Cardiac arrhythmia and conduction disorders age < 70 w/o C.C. | $500 each day for two days, $200 each day thereafter |
| 140 Angina pectoris | $750 for first day, $250 each day thereafter |

diagnostic laboratory services to physician offices. In such circumstances, the hospital's objectives typically include using excess capacity to reduce fixed costs per unit of output, increasing profits, providing diagnostic services to third-party payers under contractual arrangements, serving as a barrier-to-entry for competitors, and establishing better relationships with other providers/physicians.

For example, assume that a hospital determines that excess capacity exists in its laboratory. Furthermore, the marginal costs of its laboratory services are estimated to be only the costs of supplies actually consumed, since excess equipment and staffing (second and third shift) resources exist. By determining its marginal costs, the hospital is in a position to proactively contract for diagnostic laboratory tests with physician offices, employer health services, or third-party payers as a way of enhancing its profitability and market position.

**Pricing Summary**

In sum, effective product and procedure pricing is vital in today's competitive health care environment. The challenge and opportunity of competitive pricing can best be met with the information supplied by a cost management system—information that is timely, accurate, reliable, and flexible. Over the longer term, as competition increases, this improved information on the costs of products and procedures will help management achieve its desired objectives and results.

## PLANNING AND BUDGETING

An important factor for a hospital to achieve success is its ability to accomplish its mission and its related goals and objectives. By improving the basis on which future action plans are built, the goals and objectives of the organization—expressed as a strategic plan—can be managed and attained more readily. The information produced by a cost management system can be designed to provide the information link between strategic and operational planning decisions. In this way, the impact of strategic decisions, such as entering into a new product line, can be reflected not only in the context of increased patient volumes and revenues but also simultaneously in the amounts and types of increased (or decreased) operational resource and cost requirements to meet a different level of demand. In this section, we focus on how cost management information can improve both the hospital's strategic planning and its operational budgeting process.

### Strategic Planning

Because the strategic plan addresses the future direction of the organization, timely, accurate, and reliable information is needed to implement the plan and to monitor the progress and success in achieving its goals and objectives. The major purpose of strategic planning is to provide a clear direction for the organization and to reduce the effects of future uncertainties. Numerous authors have documented various approaches to strategic planning for the health care industry as well as for other industries, and have described the steps in the planning process. Regardless of the strategic planning approach selected, it should include these basic activities:

- preparation of a current mission statement
- definition of current product lines and strategies to serve those product lines
- evaluation of the internal consistency of current strategies
- evaluation of current positions with respect to (1) competitors, (2) market needs, and (3) future expectations concerning technological, legislative, and demographic changes
- evaluation of threats and opportunities
- development of new strategies and action steps

- implementation of the strategies
- monitoring of the action steps of the plan

The applications of information obtained from the cost management system can serve as valuable links between these basic activities. In this section, we discuss some of these linkages as they affect the strategic planning process.

### Defining and Evaluating Product Lines

The strategic planning process includes an assessment of the product lines (products or business units) that the hospital currently offers or is considering offering in the future. As we have seen, many hospitals define their product lines in terms of major diagnostic categories (MDCs) or clinical program descriptions (for example, surgery, medical, obstetrics, ambulatory care). In each case, the hospital must decide if its current definitions are responsive to its current internal organization and external demands. The more consistent the product definitions are with respect to the marketplace understanding of them and with the hospital's internal organizational structure, the easier they will be to manage.

In essence, the cost management system helps the hospital define product lines by providing contributor information. For example, reports listing revenues, volumes, and patient days for each proposed product line are obtained through the product reporting function of the cost management system. An example of how this information might appear in a product-line activity and revenue report is shown in Exhibit 10–22.

Top management, together with physicians and product-line managers, reviews this information to confirm and, when necessary, to redefine its product lines. Typically, this process results in the collapsing of product lines that were once significant or the fragmenting of product lines that have grown substantially (for example, by forming separate product lines). After a consensus on product-line definitions is reached, reports delineating the individual products within each product line are produced. Management, again with physician and product-line manager input, then confirms or adjusts the placement of each product. Finally, individual product information is used to develop the operation plan (budget) and the detailed financial statements.

To evaluate accurately each product line with respect to the level of future investment, profitability and margin information must be reviewed. For existing product lines, this information is produced through

**Exhibit 10–22** Example of a Product-Line Activity and Revenue Report

Memorial Hospital
Product-Line Activity and Revenue Report
For the Year Ended September 30, 19XX

| | Gross Revenue | | Discharges | | Patient Days | |
|---|---|---|---|---|---|---|
| Product Line | Dollars | % of Total | Number | % of Total | Number | % of Total |
| Respiratory services | $ 4,390,859 | 8.5 | 906 | 7.5 | 11,422 | 13.3 |
| Obstetric services | 3,022,612 | 5.8 | 834 | 6.9 | 2,280 | 2.7 |
| Cardiology services | 1,729,969 | 3.3 | 629 | 5.2 | 3,219 | 3.8 |
| . | . | . | . | . | . | . |
| . | . | . | . | . | . | . |
| . | . | . | . | . | . | . |
| Totals | $51,792,363 | 100% | 12,085 | 100% | 85,619 | 100% |

the cost management system's product performance reporting function. For proposed product lines, procedure resource consumption information may be obtained from external databases, or it may be created by a panel of in-house clinical professionals (for example, a task force of physicians and nurses).

Once procedure resource consumption for a proposed product or product line is determined, fixed and variable costs are attached to each procedure, extended by their procedure usage, and then summed. Gross and net revenues are reported for all product lines to provide a means of calculating margins and profitability. Exhibit 10–23 shows how cost and revenue information provided by the cost management system is brought together to determine the profitability position of each product line.

*Assessment of Market Dynamics*

To determine more precisely the potential and degree of investment for each product line, the hospital must relate operating costs to the product's market potential. In addition to determining the individual

**Exhibit 10–23** Example of a Product-Line Profitability Report

Memorial Hospital
Product-Line Profitability Report

| | | | Per-Case Averages | | | | |
| Product Line | Gross Revenue | Deductions | Net Revenue | Variable Cost | Margin | Fixed Cost | Profit (Loss) |
|---|---|---|---|---|---|---|---|
| Respiratory services | $6,185 | $498 | $5,687 | $5,022 | $665 | $410 | $255 |
| Obstetric services | 2,703 | 242 | 2,461 | 2,268 | 193 | 328 | (135) |
| Ophthalmology services[1] | 1,985 | 101 | 1,884 | 1,192 | 692 | 190 | 502 |

[1]Proposed product line, for which projected figures are estimates

market share for each product line, this requires an overall assessment of market dynamics.

The components of market dynamics are market size, market development, growth opportunities, and competition. To assess its impact on the market potential of a particular product line, each component is usually ranked low, medium, or high. For example, the size of the market for ophthalmology services may be very significant and growing in an aging metropolitan area. Therefore, the market size and growth opportunity for this product line can be rated high. Conversely, obstetric services in the same community would represent a smaller and declining market size; the market size and growth opportunity for such services would be rated low. In this situation, if one of the hospital's overall strategies is to increase the elderly community's awareness of its services, ophthalmology services may be an excellent product line to invest in and develop. Moreover, if elderly patients experience comfortable, convenient, and high-quality ophthalmology services at the hospital, they will be more likely to return for other services targeted at them, such as respiratory services.

In evaluating competitors within a product line, the organization must identify the relative market share of those offering the same product line within the hospital's service area. For example, every hospital in the community may offer obstetric services regardless of profitability levels or market potential. Though a particular hospital may not want to expand aggressively its obstetric services product line, it may still want to maintain its current market share in order to provide a comprehensive set of services that are particularly important to a particular HMO or employer.

To assess market dynamics, the hospital obtains regional and national utilization data—similar to the data used for pricing—and combines them with its own utilization data to ascertain growth or market penetration potential. Physicians can play a key role in determining market potential. They can provide insights on trends in care and alternative treatments and technologies that currently exist or may shortly become available to impact the market potential of a segment of a product line (for example, birthing clinics).

An example of a market potential activity report is presented in Exhibit 10–24. The report shows an increasing market potential for ophthalmology and obstetric services, regionally and nationally; however, it shows a declining market potential for respiratory services. Yet, if, as shown in Exhibit 10–23, respiratory services are fairly profitable for the hospital, it might want to maintain or expand its market share, despite the diminishing demand.

**Exhibit 10–24** Example of a Market Potential Activity Report

Memorial Hospital
Market Potential Activity Report

| Product Line | 19X4 Percentage of Discharges | | | 19X5 Percentage of Discharges | | | 19X6 Percentage of Discharges | | |
|---|---|---|---|---|---|---|---|---|---|
| | *National* | *Regional* | *Memorial* | *National* | *Regional* | *Memorial* | *National* | *Regional* | *Memorial* |
| Respiratory services | 6.8 | 6.9 | 7.2 | 6.7 | 6.7 | 7.4 | 6.6 | 6.4 | 7.5 |
| Obstetric services | 9.1 | 9.4 | 8.8 | 9.3 | 9.8 | 8.2 | 9.4 | 10.3 | 6.9 |
| Ophthalmology services[1] | 3.2 | 3.1 | — | 3.5 | 3.8 | — | 4.9 | 5.2 | — |

[1]New product line, for which projected figures are estimates

*Determining Market Share*

As a further step in the strategic planning process, the hospital has to focus, on a more detailed level, on its own and its competitors' market shares. Several years' data may have to be reviewed to ascertain the advance or loss in market share over time. Additionally, this review may serve as a reference point in the assessment of the effectiveness of marketing strategies or of the results of competitors' actions. An example of a product-line market share report is provided in Exhibit 10–25.

Once the profitability and market share for each product line have been determined, the hospital can position them in an evaluation matrix, as shown in Figure 10–4. In this matrix, the position of the three identified product lines is different, based on their respective market potential and profitability characteristics. As noted earlier, respiratory services show a decreasing overall demand on both a national and regional basis. However, they provide a large margin ($665 per case) and moderate profitability ($255 per case). Obstetric services demonstrate an increasing demand on both a national and regional basis. However, their margin and profitability are fairly low ($193 and $135 per case, respectively). Yet, because obstetric services may have a significant future impact on the use of other services, and because the hospital may

**Exhibit 10–25** Example of a Product-Line Market Share Report

Memorial Hospital
Product-Line Market Share Analysis Report
For the Year Ending September 30, 19XX

| | Discharges | | | | Total Market | |
| | Memorial | | Competitor A | | | |
| Product Line | Number | Market Share % | Number | Market Share % | Number | % |
|---|---|---|---|---|---|---|
| Respiratory services | 906 | 22.5 | 691 | 17.2 | 4,018 | 100 |
| Obstetric services | 834 | 13.9 | 1,322 | 22.1 | 5,987 | 100 |
| Cardiology services | 629 | 15.3 | 401 | 9.8 | 4,098 | 100 |
| Totals | 12,085 | 21.2 | 14,020 | 24.6 | 57,005 | 100 |

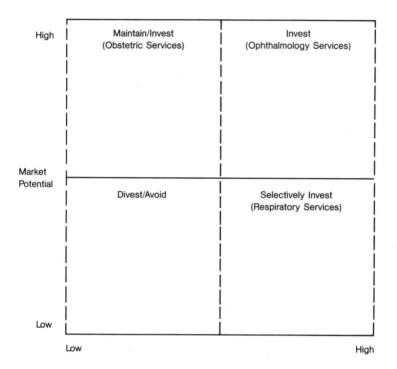

**Figure 10–4** Product-Line Evaluation Matrix

want to protect its current market share, selective investment might be advisable.

In evaluating the feasibility of developing new programs, such as ophthalmology services, a similar approach is taken. Based on national and regional utilization data, the demand for ophthalmology services has increased substantially over the past several years. Through the hospital's cost management system's cost determination function, physicians' and other health care professionals' estimates of ophthalmology procedure resource consumption can be identified and costed to arrive at margin and profitability estimates. The result of this process shows high margins and profitability per case ($692 and $502 respectively), as shown in Exhibit 10–23. Therefore, ophthalmology services appear to represent an opportunity that warrants investment, as can be seen in the Figure 10–4 matrix.

### Selecting Among Alternative Strategic Plans

Based on the positioning of its product lines, the hospital can now analyze its current situation and evaluate future options. This provides the basis for developing one or several alternative strategic plans. The final decision as to which strategy or strategies to pursue will depend on related operational and financial constraints. For example, the option to develop an ophthalmology program might be limited because trained and qualified physicians are not available. The lack of specialized personnel might also constrain the hospitals' ability to expand or develop a program. For example, specialized nursing personnel are required in the delivery of open heart surgery services. By determining the amount of nursing time required for each open heart procedure—through the procedure standard-setting process—a cost management system forecast of nursing full-time equivalents (FTEs) required for future years can be determined. As the product line progresses toward its targeted activity, the hospital can anticipate the number of additional nurses to be hired to meet upcoming levels of demand, thus ensuring the hospital's capability to deliver the requisite services.

Another limiting factor may be an inability to deliver due to constraints in capacity. Most hospitals have excess bed capacity; however they may not have adequate equipment, space, or staff to handle increased patient volumes. A hospital may investigate opportunities to expand a certain product line, based on available profitability and demand information. However, departmental reports from the cost management system might show that an expansion of services will result in an overextension of current capacities, requiring the purchase of additional equipment, a remodeling process, or an increase in staffing levels. Due to these projections of increased expenditures in their accompanying time frames, originally anticipated profit margins may have to be reduced significantly, thereby causing a revision of strategies.

In this way, cost management information can help hospital executives to evaluate, effectively and efficiently, the effects that alternative demand assumptions and pricing strategies will have on the hospital's profitability and operations. If the decision is to go ahead with expansion, the various operational changes in the functional departments can be determined, communicated, and budgeted effectively. In any event, based on the outcomes of each demand scenario, the related decisions that are made will ultimately affect the future course of the hospital.

Financial considerations might also constrain certain strategic alternatives and actions. For example, investments in technology are typically expensive, requiring further indebtedness, significant cash outlays, or long-term rental/lease commitments. Specialized technology also may require considerable remodeling efforts to ensure an efficient and professional work environment. In such cases, due to a limitation on funds, the hospital might have to choose a strategic alternative that does not promise as much market potential/profitability as other alternatives.

### Implementing the Strategic Plan

After considering all relevant constraints, the hospital can now finalize its strategic plan and begin the implementation process. This process generally involves the setting of various business objectives—improving (relative) quality, improving efficiency, and so on—and defining the various strategies needed to achieve those objectives. (The following chapter provides an in-depth discussion of the various strategies available to hospitals to achieve their strategic and profitability objectives.)

Once the strategic plan is implemented, it has to be monitored with regard to its progress and success. Adjustments must be made in the plan and in operations in reaction to changing market factors, for example, another hospital starting a competing program, and to changes in various internal components of the plan, for example, increased physician recruitment efforts. In this process, the cost management system can provide valuable information (described in the above performance reporting section) to assess the position and progress of each product line.

## Budgeting

After the goals and objectives of the hospital are documented within the strategic plan, they become the basis for the organization's annual budget. The budget translates the strategic plan into a defined set of departmental activity expectations, revenue levels, and expenditure targets and, ultimately, into forecasted financial statements. The budget reduces the hospital's strategies to smaller components and provides each product-line and cost center manager with the information necessary to plan specific activities within the manager's sphere of influence.

An example of a departmental expense budget is shown in Exhibit 10–26. Typically, the budget covers an entire year (12 or 13 periods), includes a staffing plan, and provides a separate line for each of the significant expenses incurred by the department.

As detailed earlier in Chapter 3, the translation of volume forecasts into detailed budgeted revenues and expenses for each selected product line or cost center is accomplished by the cost management system. As the budget year progresses, changes in volume levels can be monitored,

**Exhibit 10–26** Example of a Departmental Expense Budget Report

Memorial Hospital
Departmental Budget Report
For the Year Ending September 30, 19XX

| General Ledger Account | Periods | | | | Total |
|---|---|---|---|---|---|
| | 1 | 2 | 3 | | |
| 100  Manager | $ 3,000 | $ 3,000 | $ 3,000 | | $ 36,000 |
| 200  Technician | 24,650 | 21,250 | 17,400 | | 239,200 |
| 300  Clerk | 2,800 | 2,800 | 2,800 | | 11,536 |
| 600  Office supplies | 650 | 450 | 700 | | 7,316 |
| 700  Film | 15,250 | 16,100 | 16,250 | | 180,880 |
| 800  Developer | 1,800 | 1,680 | 2,010 | | 20,642 |
| 1000 Magazines | 50 | 0 | 100 | | 410 |
| 1100 Seminars | 0 | 0 | 1,400 | | 5,000 |
| 1400 Rent | 2,000 | 2,000 | 2,000 | | 24,000 |
| 1500 Leases | 2,300 | 2,300 | 2,300 | | 28,290 |
| Totals | $52,500 | $49,580 | $47,960 | | $553,274 |

and the required adjustments to staffing and other resource utilization can be made.

A well-designed cost management system allows management to adjust the budget easily and accurately for unforeseen changes in the business environment. For example, a new third-party contract negotiated during the year may have an impact on case mix and volume. The cost management system can provide the information needed to reflect properly the impact of the new contract on the affected departmental budgets. The ability to adjust accurately to such changes and to reset performance targets accordingly provides managers with the maximum amount of latitude in their individual decision-making responsibilities. Also, the ability to adjust the budget accurately to take into account unforeseen developments maintains the budget's integrity as one means of assessing a manager's performance.

The linkage between the strategic and operational planning processes that is provided by the cost management system may also benefit the hospital by reducing the budgeting responsibilities of the department managers. This would make additional time available to concentrate on improving production and the quality of care, which in turn can lead to a more cost-efficient and quality-efficient delivery of services.

**Summary Planning and Budgeting**

Accurate, timely, and attainable plans will, in effect, chart the course of action for the entire organization. A significant portion of the information that is necessary to complete and implement these plans is derivable from a cost management system. Then, once the planning decisions have been made and the selected plans implemented, the cost management system can be used on an ongoing basis to refine departmental budgets and monitor the hospital's performance.

## SUMMARY

A cost management system produces valuable information to support the decision-making responsibilities of virtually all levels of hospital management. The types of data produced and their importance to the hospital will depend on their utility in application to specific managerial issues. The resulting benefit will be the enhanced ability of the hospital to monitor, control, and reduce its costs. This, in turn, will provide a valuable competitive advantage to the hospital.

# chapter 11

# A Strategic Cost Management Model

## INTRODUCTION

Today's health care environment has changed the rules by which hospitals can remain profitable and accomplish their mission. To remain (or become) profitable, hospitals must assess the changes in their environments and then respond to those changes in a decisive and timely manner. Top management must constantly monitor its environment, evaluate its strengths and weaknesses in responding to that environment, and assess the related potential threats and opportunities. Then, it must formulate and implement appropriate business strategies.

In this final chapter, we show how a strategic cost management model—adapted from other industries—can use cost management information to select and assign priorities in the development of business strategies to help hospitals achieve their profitability objectives.

## DEFINING THE MODEL

A strategic cost management model provides the framework for facilitating business decision making, for assigning priorities to business strategies, and, ultimately, for improving the hospital's financial position. Because the overall objective of increasing profitability is too general in nature, it is necessary to develop more specific objectives before formulating business strategies. Thus, the model enables management to organize the components of increasing profitability into distinct business objectivies. Each objective is further defined by identifying successive levels of more detailed subobjectives. Finally, business strategies are formulated to accomplish each set of objectives.

By defining and documenting business objectives in this way, management is able to formulate more carefully focused strategies. Ultimately, a well-constructed model can be used to establish a "decision tree" for developing both effective, long-term strategic decisions and short-term, tactical decisions on an ongoing basis.

### The Overall Objective: Increasing Profitability

The current health care environment places tremendous downward pressures on hospital revenues. Inpatient volumes are generally down as a result of competition, changing payment systems, expansion of managed care, employer reductions and/or control of benefits, and economic incentives for beneficiaries who seek care in a less costly setting. Price or rate per unit of care delivered is impacted by increased discounting and competitive bidding activities by payers and providers alike.

The combined effect of these downward pressures is to create substantial risks for hospitals—risks that ultimately pass through to creditors, bond holders, employees, and the community. If these risks are not addressed effectively, profitability may decrease and the hospital may not be able to achieve its mission. The inevitable response to increased risk is to accumulate more substantial equity contributions. Yet, the downward pressures on revenue and the tax law changes that challenge continued philanthropy constrain hospitals' efforts in accumulating equity. To resolve the dilemma, hospitals must generate increased equity from operations, which in turn requires them to adopt effective business strategies. In this situation, cost management information, incorporated as an integral component of the strategic planning process, can help management evaluate and select the appropriate business strategies and to monitor and control the strategies implemented.

Many factors affect a hospital's profit requirements. For example, an investor-owned hospital might pursue an expected return on investment to fulfill obligations to investors, in addition to providing high-quality services to the community. A free-standing rural hospital may be more concerned about how it can provide comprehensive services to its community. Another relevant factor is philanthropy. Some hospitals receive generous philanthropic gifts or have significant income-producing endowments—providing them with a "safety net" for the future. Whatever the income circumstance or factors that affect a specific institution, increasing profitability can enable it to accumulate the resources necessary to maintain current programs and to establish sufficient equity for sustained future growth.

## Setting Objectives

In addressing the overall profitability issue in the context of a strategic cost management model, four common hospital profitability objectives can be identified:

1. increasing (relative) market share
2. improving productivity
3. improving (relative) quality
4. improving fiscal management

Each of these objectives arises from a different perspective of the hospital organization. Increasing relative market share relates to the hospital's external position as a competitor in the health care marketplace. Improving productivity concerns the internal organization and its efficiency. Improving relative quality has to do with the effectiveness and perceptions of care provided to patients. Finally, improving fiscal management relates to the hospital's business function.

Although these objectives do not constitute an exhaustive list, they can serve as a framework to highlight a number of different business strategies. As the accomplishment of these objectives changes in relation to historical levels, so does the hospital's profitability. The hospital thus must identify, analyze, and implement the appropriate business strategies to achieve the objectives it has established, with the ultimate goal of establishing greater control over profitability levels.

The progress a hospital achieves toward its profitability objectives often depends on how responsive it is to the environment in which it operates. An institution's ability to respond decisively and quickly is largely a result of knowing its strengths and weaknesses in relation to threats and opportunities arising from changes in the environment. These threats and opportunities are usually classified as either internal or external:

- Internal threats and opportunities typically involve the areas of quality, productivity, and financial management. They are generally recognized by reviewing information relating to cost management, quality assurance/utilization, and financial reporting. For example, performance reports from the cost management system may show that ancillary cost center productivity is substantially below planned levels. If this situation is allowed to continue, the hospital's profitability would undoubtedly suffer. Supplemental comparative data from commercial databases, governmental agencies, and professional organizations also can help hospitals recognize, confirm, and deal with internal threats and opportunities.

- External threats and opportunities are typically related to market share issues. They may involve new competitors (for example, physicians), expansion opportunities related to service contracting, the launching of new services, or changes in the demographics of the community. Information regarding market factors, such as absolute demand, is critical in recognizing and qualifying external threats and opportunities. For example, the hospital's cost management system may report that pediatric services are profitable. This could indicate an opportunity to expand pediatric services to increase profits. However, by examining demand data, the hospital may determine that the opportunity is limited, due to an aging population or changes in competitor capabilities.

In response to these internal and external threats and opportunities, the hospital's business strategies and the impact of those strategies on profitability will establish the overall strategic direction of the hospital.

In Table 11–1, we present a generic hospital strategic cost management model. The model's profit potential column permits the hospital to assign priorities to each of its selected strategies. In the remainder of this chapter, we profile the alternative business strategies that may be selected in this model. It should be emphasized here that the model is a simple generic framework; each hospital must design and evaluate its own model to ensure that it reflects its unique needs and objectives.

**Table 11–1**  A Strategic Cost Management Model

| Overall Objective | Objectives | Business Strategies | Profit Potential | Hospital-Specific Strategies |
|---|---|---|---|---|
| Increasing Profitability | Increasing (Relative) Market Share | Merger and Acquisition | | |
| | | Marketing | | |
| | Improving Productivity | Clinical Efficiency | | |
| | | Operations Efficiency | | |
| | Improving (Relative) Quality | Diagnosis and Treatment Planning | | |
| | | Patient Satisfaction | | |
| | Improving Fiscal Management | Fixed Capital | | |
| | | Cash Management | | |

## FOUR BASIC OBJECTIVES

### Increasing (Relative) Market Share

Decreasing demand in many communities, especially for inpatient services, has resulted in hospitals trying to increase their market share as a means of improving or maintaining their profitability levels. For example, maintaining or increasing volume is effective in leveraging a hospital's fixed-cost base or excess capacity. Thus, it is understandable that the health care industry has placed its greatest emphasis on obtaining additional patient volumes. Indeed, for many hospitals, this has become the dominant competitive issue.

To ensure a positive profitability impact, it is essential that both anticipated revenue and the associated costs are quantified during the strategic planning process. More volume is generally better, but more volume also has its costs. Unless profitability is reasonably estimated, incorrect decisions in relation to competing market share options may result. Two business strategies—merger/acquisition and marketing—are commonly used to increase market share and profitability selectively.

#### *Merger/Acquisition*

The merger/acquisition of established health care facilities—other hospitals, physician practices, clinics, managed-care organizations, and so on—may enhance a hospital's ability to expand market share. Mergers and acquisitions can be characterized as either horizontal or vertical integrations. While many organizations have combined horizontal and vertical entities, the anticipated outcome is generally the same: to enhance market share selectively and provide a more comprehensive product offering.

**Horizontal Merger/Acquisition.** Historically, the dominant feature of horizontal acquisition has been the expansion by the main organization into other geographic territories. In many combinations of this type, the principal purpose was to leverage the profitability of existing facilities. A second but less important purpose was to develop an integrated health care delivery network that would be more cost-effective and produce higher-quality care. The initial growth of many investor-owned systems has been characterized by horizontal acquisitions.

In recent years, combination activities increasingly have involved the development of feeder/hub networks of facilities. The following are major advantages of establishing a feeder/hub network through horizontal acquisition:

- *Improved resource allocation.* Redundant, expensive, or capital-intensive services, such as imaging services, may be reduced by having one facility offer a service and receive transfers/referrals from other affiliated facilities.
- *Expanded market distribution channels.* These provide convenience features for employers whose employees are dispersed throughout several communities. Expanded versions of such channels are being tested nationally through such alternative non-ownership relationships as Voluntary Hospitals of America, American Healthcare System, and Premier Hospitals Alliance, Inc.
- *Improved management skills and retention.* Multifacility organizations often provide executives and middle managers with continued career growth within the organization. This helps the organizations attract and retain highly qualified and motivated professionals, including physicians.

**Vertical Merger/Acquisition.** A strategy that employs vertical acquisition recognizes that a patient's health care needs begin prior to admission and extend beyond discharge. Also, it recognizes that major developments in health care technology are resulting in reduced (or alternatives to) inpatient stays. Accordingly, many hospitals are developing pre- and post-inpatient provider care capabilities. Patients may leave the hospital earlier, but they do not necessarily leave the health care system. An increasingly large number of hospitals are providing remote ambulatory care facilities, clinics, subacute inpatient care services, and home health care services. By making such services available to the patient within the hospital's network before or after a hospital stay, a broad continuum of services can be provided. This type of vertical integration strategy provides several benefits:

- *A comprehensive package of services.* The packaging of services results in a total health care system, not just medical care. It also facilitates contracting, since multiple levels of care can be contracted with one organization. This generally leads to improved flexibility, reduced costs, and improved cash flow.
- *Maximization of revenue per patient.* The organization is able to provide many different types and levels of health care services, thereby keeping patient revenue within its network.

- *Economies of scale.* A large organization can achieve many economies of scale, such as reduced marketing costs, group purchasing,
  and reduced personnel costs.

Vertical integration may extend beyond providing services to include
undertaking insurance risk. By creating hospital-based health maintenance organizations, developing preferred provider arrangements, and
accepting per-capita payments, the hospital can assume the actuarial
risks of an insurer. Sufficient history does not exist to evaluate the
effectiveness of vertical integration into insurance markets. However,
several early attempts by major provider organizations have met with
difficulty. Since insurance and provider industries are basically different enterprises, barriers to complete integration often exist. The barriers usually involve the initial intense capitalization requirements,
higher levels of risk, and specialized talent requirements inherent in the
insurance industry.

**The Cost Management Role.** Cost management information enables
health care executives to make better informed decisions regarding
market share strategies in merger/acquisitions. For example, it can be
used to examine the profitability of the hospital's various product lines
and to determine areas of excess capacity, such as operating suites or
rehabilitation facilities. Then, efforts to pursue more profitable product
lines through mergers or acquisitions or in ventures with physician
groups can provide all parties with a mutually advantageous arrangement, resulting in better use of the hospital's physical plant and better
means of attracting patients to high-quality facilities and providers.

Indeed, cost management information is often essential to determine
appropriate staffing increases or reductions associated with duplicate
services following an acquisition or merger. For example, volume
increases may result in capacity constraints in some cost centers.
Through its flexible budgeting capabilities, a cost management system
can determine additional staffing levels, accurately based on alternative
demand scenarios. Conversely, staffing reductions may be determined
more effectively and accurately through use of a cost management
system. Finally since market share strategies are an ongoing process,
not a one-time undertaking, cost management information can provide
the basis for the continuous monitoring of the profitability of each
segment of a complex health care organization, compared with expectations.

*Marketing*

The marketing of health care services has evolved steadily during the
1980s to correspond with changes in the health care environment. In

years past, public relations and fund development were the mainstays of health care marketing. Today, the activities associated with marketing range from product-specific advertising, to pricing promotions and direct sales/contracting activities. Not only has the product focus changed, the targeted channels for patients now include payers/insurers, employers, and physicians, in addition to the consumer.

Ultimately, employers and insurers seek cost-effective health care at acceptable levels of quality and convenience. Quality of care and convenience cannot yet be evaluated objectively, but they can be used as subjective thresholds in evaluating options.

Price is currently a major factor in the evaluation of alternative provider contracts. In a price-competitive environment, value added in the form of additional services may result in a competitive advantage for the hospital. For instance, employers that administer their own insurance plans may benefit from a single comprehensive provider by reducing claims handling costs.

To attract physicians, hospitals must use a different marketing approach. Program sophistication, staff ability, technology level, and convenience are important attributes that will enhance a physician's career potential. Also, a favorable image is important in attracting good physicians. In short, a hospital or health care provider should emphasize those attributes that are likely to benefit physicians and reconsider other attributes that represent threats to them.

The hospital's image also often influences its profitability. Maintaining a good image requires not only the provision of high-quality services; it also requires the promotion of the perception of high-quality services within the community. Patients see a hospital's heart transplant program on a local television news program and assume that all of the hospital's programs are equally advanced. Yet, being the first hospital in a service area to offer a new technology is only one way to foster the perception of high quality. A spinoff perception of advanced services and technology at teaching or tertiary care facilities often elevates its core services to a similar high-quality status.

Public relations and advertising campaigns are useful in extending the perception of quality. Often, however, it is difficult to draw a clear distinction between actual and perceived quality. Most hospitals promote a vision of themselves as high-quality, clinically and technologically advanced providers of health care. But, it is becoming clear that the promotion of a perception of quality must also have some foundation in fact—a unique program, a special capability, or some distinctive competency that sets the hospital apart.

Marketing actions as a response to competition, by providers and purchasers alike, often focus on price preferences through discounting. Some providers position themselves as unique, high-quality providers. Generally, the American public values the availability of high-quality health care services more than the advantage of paying the lowest price for services, particularly since consumers often do not pay directly for the services rendered.

The growing competition with respect to price, quality, and convenience means that many hospitals must reevaluate their role in the health care delivery system. Increased networking and contracting enables many hospitals to address market segments separately. Concentration or de-emphasis may occur selectively for products, payers, geographic areas, or other market segments. Efforts and resources may be directed primarily toward the areas of highest marginal return (on both a per-unit and total basis).

Cost management information provides management with a tool for determining the areas with the greatest marketing potential. It enables top management to target market segments—payers, physicians, products, and locations—that will provide the greatest profitability potential. Once these segments have been identified, the cost management system can provide the information needed to evaluate pricing and investment options effectively and to monitor follow-up performance.

**Improving Productivity**

When third-party payers utilized cost-based reimbursement mechanisms, the financial impact of improvements in productivity was greatly diluted. As hospitals increasingly assume more risk for the services they provide, the incentives for identifying and implementing productivity improvements have become more critical.

The current trend of the health care environment—fixed fee and capitation payments—enables hospitals to retain more of their savings from productivity improvements. Not surprisingly, then, there has been a new emphasis on efforts in productivity improvement. These efforts have been directed at two areas of productivity: clinical efficiency and operational efficiency.

*Clinical Efficiency*

Clinical efficiency is a measure of how well physicians/clinicians conform to the clinical practice protocol developed by their peers. The research and evaluation involved in establishing treatment protocols is intended not only to ensure quality but also to define clinical efficiency. However, there are clear cautions to be noted when dealing with clinical efficiency—particularly since there is some "art" to medicine, it is not all science.

The quality assurance and utilization review activities that monitor compliance often result in more streamlined treatments and in improved quality and efficiency. Vertical integration into alternative facilities and programs also promotes clinical efficiency, by providing the proper level of care in the most cost-effective setting.

By providing detailed historical treatment profiles, cost management information systems can provide input into the development of strategies for identifying protocols development and improving clinical efficiency. The profiles provide a tool that physicians can use to analyze and improve the quality and cost-effectiveness of treatment.

Accurate cost information is essential in the implementation of this strategy. First, it identifies those products that are high in cost. This helps to focus attention on those products that have the greatest potential to realize cost savings. Second, it quantifies the amount of savings that may be expected by addressing atypical treatment regimens and showing where to expend educational or other resources to influence physician behavior patterns.

For example, Swan-Ganz catheter insertions are fairly routine in intensive care units; in a 10-bed ICU, three to five patients, on average, have Swan-Ganz catheters in place. Each catheter costs about $150, not including the insertion kits or other supplies required to place the catheter. Proper placement of the catheter requires that its tip be easily advanced into the pulmonary artery. Because of poor technique or inexperience, several attempts may be necessary to place the catheter. Also, during insertion, the catheter can easily become contaminated, or blood clots that cannot be flushed from the catheter may form. Therefore, it is not uncommon for two to three catheters to be used per placement attempt. Once inserted, an x-ray verifies that the tip of the catheter is in the pulmonary artery and that a pneumothorax has not occurred. If a pneumothorax does occur, a longer, more intensive stay is generally required.

By recognizing and quantifying the magnitude of this catheter problem, the hospital can determine and implement solutions that not only reduce costs but that also improve the quality of care. Practical solutions may include increased in-service education, the use of a specific skilled nurse or IV team that is responsible for the insertion of the Swan-Ganz catheters, or the availability of an in-house physician specialist. If 500 patients required a Swan-Ganz catheter and catheter usage were reduced on average by one per patient, the annual savings would be $75,000. In addition, the cost management system could report the amount of costs saved in other areas, due to a decrease in the incidents of pneumothoracies.

Treatment variances reported by the cost management system can provide an ongoing means of assisting physician and product-line managers in formulating and implementing product-line business strategies. The investigation into the causes of treatment variances will identify the level of compliance with treatment planning standards determined in the protocol, as well as the variations in actual treatment patterns.

For example, the standard resource utilization for a product-specific treatment is based on all such treatments over a period of time. The examination of product-specific treatment variances by individual physicians may suggest that certain physicians are obtaining successful results by using more cost-effective treatment programs. Usually a more thorough study of the characteristics of the patients treated and the results obtained are required to support or refute this initial interpretation.

Product resource consumption standards that are established without consideration of treatment differences due to patient severity produce incrementally less favorable variances for the physician who is managing the most severe cases. For instance, because of a favorable reputation, a cardiologist may receive referrals of only the most difficult cases. The resources necessary to treat these patients is typically in excess of that necessary to treat less acutely ill cardiology patients. Unless further investigations are undertaken, the dissimilarity in patient characteristics may result in an inaccurate evaluation of the quality and cost-effectiveness of the medical treatment provided.

## Operational Efficiency

A second business strategy to accomplish the productivity improvement objective is to improve the efficiency of functional cost centers, thereby reducing the unit cost of services. The application of cost management is most closely associated with increased operational efficiency. As previously discussed, the procedural standard-setting process and the ongoing review of results together will identify many opportunities to improve operational efficiency. This type of inward look at the hospital's operations can in turn produce significant profitability gains for the hospital. Three components of operational efficiency—systems improvement, human resource enhancement, and automation—are typically addressed as tactics to improve productivity.

**Systems Improvement.** By addressing systems improvement, numerous opportunities can be identified to reduce costs—and ultimately improve productivity. One way to improve interdepartmental relationships and reduce overhead and managerial costs is through organizational resizing. For example, assume a hospital has separate managers for its occupational, physical, and speech therapy cost centers. Through a strategic resizing analysis, it may be determined that only a single manager is needed to coordinate the activities of the three areas. Not only does this change reduce hospital costs by reducing personnel, it can also help the hospital achieve or maintain a competitive cost advantage, by improving the attractiveness of the hospital in the marketplace. Other systems improvements may include altering physical layouts, improving staffing and scheduling policies and procedures, and simplifying or automating work processes to reduce labor requirements. In all these situations, information from a cost management system can be used to identify the areas where improvement may be needed and to quantify the savings expected from system improvement activities. Then the system's performance reporting capabilities can be utilized to monitor the progress toward achieving expected or targeted savings levels over time.

**Human Resource Enhancement.** Here, the focus is not on the amount of labor hours consumed, but rather on the additional value to be realized in comparison with the additional costs incurred. The goal of human resource enhancement is to improve employee capabilities and skills through education, management development, and other motivational and behavior modifications. This usually leads to higher-quality services and, possibly, to reduced staffing levels. Similarly, morale and retention may be monitored and optimized to ensure a supply of skilled labor, thereby possibly reducing recruiting and personnel costs.

**Automation.** Procedural standard setting generally provides the information necessary to evaluate the cost-effectiveness of placing new technology into the production process. Many opportunities exist to improve efficiency through the automation of diagnostic and therapeutic procedures, as well as clerical functions. The anticipated trade-off for increased technological investment is reduced staffing, improved quality, and enhanced delivery capabilities. For example, to improve efficiency and quality in its diagnostic x-ray department, a hospital might install automatic film developers. As the learning curve for this new equipment decreases, operational efficiencies and cost savings result in the form of reduced staffing and less film spoilage.

Improvements in technology are not limited to the clinical areas of the hospital. For example, advanced word processing equipment may be used to reduce medical record transcription time and cost per patient record. Similarly, automation or technology may be inserted into information flow networks, such as order-entry results reporting or other patient care systems. Like other types of technology, information flow networks reduce human effort, expedite the flow of critical information, increase productivity, and improve delivery capabilities—often leading to higher quality and lower costs.

Yet, while technology can provide myriad benefits, caution should be exercised by the hospital when weighing the cost benefits of technology options. Though advanced technology can often provide operational efficiencies and higher quality, it also tends to be expensive. Also, more advanced equipment typically requires a more skilled workforce. In addition, many equipment vendors require that the hospital use their supplies, thereby eliminating cost savings derived through group purchasing arrangements or multiple competing vendors. Finally, in addition to the purchase or lease/rent price of equipment, the hospital may have long-term maintenance contracts to consider. In all these situations, the hospital must examine its cash position, since capital expenditures generally require a substantial outlay of cash at a specific point in time.

Another key component to be considered in automation is the capacity of the new technology. The fixed per-unit cost portion of procedures is dependent on total fixed costs divided by total procedure volumes. Therefore, if an activity is not increased, or at least maintained at a minimum, costs per unit of output for newer more expensive technology will increase substantially. This type of information, available from the cost management system, can be used as one criterion when selecting among technologies that have varying levels of capacity limits and related prices.

Cost management information can also be used to estimate the trade-offs between advanced technology improvements in current operations. In this way, by assessing the overall impact potential automation changes have on the cost of services, both variable costs (personnel and supplies) and fixed costs (base equipment and maintenance contract costs) per unit of output can be managed better.

**Improving Relative Quality**

Cost-based reimbursement systems tend to minimize the impact that quality has on profitability. Essentially, these payment mechanisms link payments to inputs rather than outputs. Consequently, revenue and profitability may be increased by excess utilization, which does not necessarily translate into higher-quality care. For example, most hospital managers and physicians would agree that long preoperative or recuperative stays may be indicators of excess utilization, and perhaps of a poor quality of care (for example, more opportunity for infections and other hospital-caused problems). Yet, this overutilization of services would be economically rewarded by many payment mechanisms.

Quality is related to the planned, actual, and perceived effectiveness of the treatment provided to the patient. While planned, actual, and perceived effectiveness of treatment is not easy to measure, quality is becoming an important factor in differentiating services, and it is likely ultimately to influence a hospital's long-term survival. Hospitals that demonstrate poor quality care often receive adverse publicity and more malpractice claims and are subject to other detrimental actions. Conversely, hospitals that are involved in sophisticated activities—such as heart transplant operations—are often perceived as high-quality providers, resulting in enhanced volumes and income.

Thus, assuming that quality is a relatively high priority, hospitals may enhance profitability by increasing the relative quality of services they offer. With quality improvement as the objective, the hospital's business strategies should be directed toward diagnosis and treatment planning and toward patient satisfaction, as indicated in Table 11–1.

*Diagnosis and Treatment Planning*

Whereas treatment efficiency compares actual and planned delivery of services, diagnosis and treatment planning focuses on the "planned" methods of delivering patient care in order to identify proven and effective treatment options. Treatment planning includes protocol development, technology training and development, and logistics planning. Cost management systems will provide the base of historical clinical and demographic patient/product data needed to challenge critical treatment planning issues.

**Protocols.** The diagnosis and treatment of an individual patient is generally directed by the patient's physician, with input from other physicians, nurses, therapists, and health care professionals. A physician's treatment protocol in a given situation has historically been based on the physician's clinical training and experience. The resulting utilization of services to treat the patient was rarely questioned or evaluated. The advent of Medicare's Prospective Payment System and the increased market share gained by managed care arrangements signals a critical need to review resource utilization.

Again, the hospital's cost management system is a critical component of the effort. The system can report resource consumption at a patient level to permit comparative analyses and to assist physicians to define, manage, and challenge treatment regimens based on those analyses. Protocols establish benchmarks for evaluating resource consumption that is atypical. They also may be used as a basis for evaluating alternative treatments to achieve improved quality and delivery of treatment. By carefully reviewing existing treatment practices, a dialogue concerning the critical variables in the diagnostic or treatment process can be created. By capitalizing on that dialogue, through challenges and education, the hospital can bring about significant cost reductions and quality-of-care improvements.

The cost management system also serves as a basis for asking clinical questions about historical results. This serves to enhance quality and consistency in the patient care process. The end result of higher quality, more cost-effective care will ultimately influence the hospital's profitability objectives.

**Technology.** In addition to its positive impact on clinical efficiency and productivity as noted earlier, the introduction of technology often impacts on the quality of patient care. Computerized tomography (CT) scanning and magnetic resonance imaging (MRI) are two high-technology tools that often lead to faster and more accurate diagnoses. The resulting improvement in the diagnostic process may in turn hasten the implementation of the appropriate treatment—again leading to higher quality and improved cost-effectiveness. Similarly, the lithotripter and balloon angioplasty are often cited as examples of technology's favorable impact on treatment and the subsequent recovery process. Thus, though often costly, technology may, by minimizing risks, be a cost-justified means of improving quality. Additionally, it may reduce the consumption of other resources (for example, nursing services), thereby lowering the overall cost of care.

**Logistics.** For hospitals, logistics represents the relationship and location of the various resources and departments required in the patient care process. For example, the existence of a central database of patient clinical, status, and location information can improve the treatment process. This logistical arrangement is similar to that of the assembly process in manufacturing companies. People, parts, and technology must be available at specific points in time to produce high-quality outputs economically and effectively. In the hospital, the coordination of scheduling between ancillary and nursing departments ensures that patients are properly prepared and available for upcoming treatments, thereby minimizing cancellations. The logistics of patient care is thus an important component of efficient operations, and it is especially important to the patient's perception of quality care.

For example, logistics can positively impact quality through reduced waiting time for specimen pick-up and results reporting or in the ready availability of key supplies or pharmaceuticals. In these instances, not only is quality improved, but fewer staff may be required, since delays and waiting times are reduced. If tests are batched for processing (for example, diagnostic laboratory tests), fewer supplies (controls and standards) are used and more specimens can be processed at a single time, thereby reducing costs without altering quality. If supplies or key personnel (for example, an anesthesiologist) are available, the treatment process usually progresses more smoothly. Conversely, if the absence of those supplies or personnel is discovered only hours or minutes before a surgical procedure, delays in the treatment of the patient and the idle time of valuable surgical suites is increased, thereby increasing costs—not to mention the adverse impact on the patient.

Continuous monitoring must take place to ensure that logistic improvements are cost- and quality-effective. Cost management information provides management with the tools to determine proper levels of people, supplies, and technology to administer both high-quality and cost-effective services. These tools include staffing utilization reports, economic-order-quantities of supplies, and equipment utilization reports.

For example, the emergency department requires that supplies, personnel, and equipment of many varieties be readily available to meet a normally unknown type and volume of activity. If the supply of available resources greatly exceeds their usage over a period of time, the hospital's emergency room may become quality-effective, but highly cost-ineffective. Obviously, no hospital or community can afford to continue in this manner for long, because profitability will suffer and funds will be unnecessarily diverted from other programs. For the emergency department to be both cost- and quality-effective, proper levels of resources need to be determined and continually managed.

*Patient Satisfaction*

Patient satisfaction is the nonclinical component of quality. Patient satisfaction is related to the process of patient care and its related perceptions, not necessarily to the outcome of treatment. It involves the overall impression the hospital makes on the patient. A positive impression enhances the likelihood that the individual will select the hospital for future health care services and perhaps influence other potential patients toward the same decision. While positive impressions obviously can have a favorable impact on the hospital, negative impressions can have serious unfavorable impacts, causing the hospital's financial position to suffer through slower payment, adverse publicity, and reduced volume.

Numerous factors can affect the patient's impression of the hospital: interactions with hospital staff, the hospital environment, the logistics of the patient stay and overall attitudes presented to the patient.

The interactions between the staff and patients probably have the greatest impact on patient satisfaction. A patient who receives personal attention gets the impression of receiving special treatment. Interestingly, most personal attention does not require more time by employees, rather, it requires more thought. Addressing the patient by name, smiling, and showing genuine concern all communicate special attention. These uses of interpersonal skills require communication and commitment by management, and perhaps additional training and education.

The environment includes the physical appearance of the facility, its furnishings, and their upkeep. This is what the patient sees and touches. Dirty hallways and cold meals can quickly create patient dissatisfaction. On the other hand, significant improvements in the patient's environment, while incurring additional costs, may have a positive overall cost benefit.

Careful control of patient care logistics will also improve a patient's impression of care at the hospital. Patient satisfaction can be enhanced by reducing waiting time in ancillary departments, emphasizing physician and staff communication, and facilitating smooth admission and discharge policies. For example, if the patient's diagnostic x-rays are performed with minimal or no waiting time, the patient probably will perceive the hospital as a high-quality, efficiently run organization. Conversely, if left unattended in a hallway waiting for treatment, the patient will probably experience some level of uneasiness and a corresponding perception of disorganization, indifference, and low-quality care on the part of the hospital and its staff. Often, the logistics of patient care is even more critical in outpatient areas, where patients may have a greater choice of where they want to be treated.

In all these situations, unfavorable patient satisfaction presents a barrier toward progress in increasing or maintaining volumes. While favorable patient satisfaction may not result in increased short-term referrals to a facility, unfavorable patient impressions may result in referrals away from the facility, constraining the hospital's ability to achieve its profitability objectives.

## Improving Fiscal Management

The fourth objective that a hospital should pursue in its strategic cost management model is to improve profitability through better fiscal management. Traditional business strategies to achieve this objective differ widely, due to the mixed nature of payment systems in the health care industry. However, business strategies that focus on reducing fixed capital expenditures and improving cash management may be implemented independently of the payment mechanisms in place, without incurring significant additional costs.

### Capital Expenditures

Aggressive capital management—either increasing the utilization of existing capacity or increasing the average age of the hospital's plant—can improve profitability. Capacity utilization is generally increased by increasing market share. Volume increases may come from traditional (horizontal) services, from vertical integration, or from nonhealth care services (for example, day care, retail shops, etc.). In some instances, capacity utilization may be increased by reducing capacity (for example, by selling a portion of the hospital's physical plant). However, unlike that of a manufacturer with several plants, a hospital's capacity is generally indivisible in nature. Therefore, capacity reductions may be limited to the elimination of off-campus sites or the disposition of major movable equipment.

A second way to reduce fixed capital expenses is to allow the average age of the plant to increase. By delaying the purchase of replacement assets and allowing assets to become debt-free or fully depreciated, profitability can be improved and cash reserves can be increased. However, there are possible drawbacks to this approach, including increased maintenance costs, a perceived decline in the relative quality of services, or a less favorable image.

## Cash Management

By minimizing noncash current assets and maximizing noninterest bearing current liabilities, hospitals can increase their available cash, thereby increasing their income-earning investments. Probably the best strategy for cash management improvement is to decrease the accounts receivable collection period. This can be accomplished by making improvements in the two phases of the collection process: billing and receipt of payment.

To improve the billing process, the hospital must first analyze the documentation required to produce a bill. By analyzing the collection and processing of the data for the documentation, constraints can be identified. Action plans to eliminate constraints can then be formulated and executed. Improving this aspect of the billing process requires a commitment from both hospital employees and physicians. Also, new data-processing systems may be needed to upgrade or augment existing capabilities. In any event, the performance of the improvements should be monitored and followed up to eliminate future problems.

The second component, receipt of payment, can be followed up in much the same way. For example, the credit and collection department must be able to identify and respond to delinquent accounts on a timely basis and to address promptly any collection difficulties encountered on specific private or third-party payer accounts. By reducing the overall accounts receivable collection period, immediate improvements in cash flow will result, thereby increasing available working capital.

Other ways to improve cash flows involve controlling the amount of prepaid expenses. Advance payments should be made only if necessary (for example, for liability insurance). Inventory supply levels may be controlled more efficiently and cash may be conserved by the introduction of better materials management procedures. Procedure standard resource and cost profiles can be used to forecast inventory item usage and to calculate accurate economic order quantities and reorder points. Finally, the maximization of current liabilities can increase income-earning investments. This is most readily done by extending the payment period on accounts payable to a reasonable limit for each vendor, without interfering with the hospital's supply channels.

In sum, the competitive nature of the health care industry, particularly of hospitals, requires that all avenues of profitability improvement be explored. Although it may not generate immediate or dramatic results, the process of improving fiscal management can provide steady incremental improvements in profitability.

## IMPLEMENTING THE MODEL

In the previous sections, we described in general terms the components of a generic strategic cost management model. To ensure the successful implementation of such a model, it is extremely important that it be designed to conform to the hospital's particular environment and situation. Each hospital must determine its own specific objectives individually. For some hospitals, the objectives we have defined in our generic model may be sufficient. Other hospitals may need to specify more objectives and to expand the model to a more detailed level. The process of combining objectives with business strategies typically results in a comprehensive "decision-tree" framework as a basis for actions.

Thus, to identify adequate specific objectives, the hospital first has to identify and qualify potential threats and opportunities. The success of this process will be directly related to the information that is available. After identifying the hospital's threats and opportunities, the specific objectives can be set. If these objectives are not carefully researched and documented, the business strategies devised to deal with the threats and opportunities will often be unfocused and ineffective. It will also be difficult to measure the progress the hospital is making in dealing with those threats and opportunities, that is to determine what a sufficient progress level is.

Once the specific objectives are determined, they should be assigned priorities based on their estimated impact on improved profitability for the hospital. Those objectives with the greatest potential to improve the hospital's current profitability position should be given the greatest emphasis.

Next, the strategies to achieve the objectives should be evaluated either as strategies for business improvement (offensive) or as strategies to avoid business risk (defensive). Here, a critical factor, especially in the case of offensive strategies, is the magnitude of impact. Those strategies that promise the greatest potential favorable impact on the organization are obviously preferable. In the case of defensive strategies, the magnitude of risk is an especially critical factor. Strategies that eliminate the greatest business risk (for example, loss of relative market share) are clearly more beneficial and should, therefore, have a higher priority in implementation.

In either case—offensive or defensive strategies—the paramount factor is the probability of success. Without a relatively high probability of success, to be selected for implementation, an option must have the potential to produce considerable benefits with a relatively low investment.

Once the strategies and their order of implementation are determined, detailed action plans should be developed. In most cases, the information from the cost management system that was used to quantify the magnitude of risk can help to identify the specific action plans needed to carry out the strategies selected for implementation.

This implementation approach enables a hospital to design its own strategic cost management model adapted to its unique situation and needs. In each case, however, to ensure optimal use of the model in the process of choosing among alternative business strategies and action plans, existing relevant constraints and success factors have to be taken into consideration. These include the availability of resources, the level of investment, and the urgency to act and react to a specific threat or opportunity.

## SUMMARY

Cost management information is essential in both the definition and the implementation phases of developing a strategic cost management model. A well-designed and well-maintained cost management system will:

- alert management to potential business threats and opportunities on a timely basis
- provide support for customizing the strategic cost management model to the specific hospital environment
- produce information as a basis for selecting the most beneficial business strategy options
- aid in monitoring the performance of the implemented options.

# Bibliography

Child, John. *Organizaton.* New York: Harper & Row, 1977.

Daft, Richard L. *Organization Theory and Design,* 4th ed. St. Paul:West Publishing Company, 1985.

Ernst & Whinney. *Health Care Joint Ventures: Survey Results.*Cleveland:author, 1985.

Haddrill, Richard M., and Moyer, John E. "Incentive Plans That Fit."*Ernst & Whinney ideas* (Fall/Winter 1985–1986):21–23.

Nackel, John G., and Kues, Irvin W. "Product-Line Management: Systems and Strategies." *Hospital and Health Services Administration* (March/April 1986):109–123.

Matz, Adolph, and Usry, Milton F. *Cost Accounting—Planning and Control.* Cincinnati, Ohio: Southwestern Publishing Co., 1980.

Sprouse, Robert T., and Moonitz, Maurice. *A Tentative Set of Broad Accounting Principles for Business Enterprises,* Accounting Research Study No. 3. New York:American Institute of Certified Public Accountants, 1962.

"Report of the Committee on Cost Concepts and Standards." *Accounting Review* 27, 1952.

# Index

*Note:* Pages appearing in italics indicate entries found in artwork.